Essays in Fundamental Immunology : 1

Essays in Fundamental Immunology : 1

EDITED BY IVAN ROITT MA, DSc(Oxon), MRCPath
Professor and Head of Department of Immunology
Middlesex Hospital Medical School, London W1

BLACKWELL SCIENTIFIC PUBLICATIONS
OXFORD LONDON EDINBURGH MELBOURNE

© 1973 Blackwell Scientific Publications
Osney Mead, Oxford
3 Nottingham Street, London W1
9 Forrest Road, Edinburgh
P.O. Box 9, North Balwyn, Victoria, Australia

All rights reserved. No part of this publication
may be reproduced, stored in a retrieval system,
or transmitted, in any form or by any means,
electronic, mechanical, photocopying, recording
or otherwise without the prior permission of
the copyright owner.

ISBN 0 632 09920 8

First published 1973

Distributed in the U.S.A. by
F.A.Davis Company, 1915 Arch Street
Philadelphia, Pennsylvania

Printed and bound in Great Britain by
Adlard & Son Ltd,
Bartholomew Press, Dorking

Contents

Preface *vi*

1 The active sites of immunoglobulin molecules *1*
   R. G. Q. LESLIE AND S. COHEN

2 The cellular and molecular basis of immunological tolerance *28*
   G. J. V. NOSSAL

3 A cellular basis for auto-immunity *44*
   J. H. L. PLAYFAIR

4 Tumour immunology *57*
   N. A. MITCHISON

Preface

This series is intended to provide a forum for the expression of ideas and perspectives in current immunological thought. The articles are aimed at undergraduates, teachers and research workers with some background in immunology. The accent is on providing lively, readable, and thought-provoking essays on selected aspects of the subject. They are not necessarily intended to be comprehensive in nature but for those determined to read further, a number of references are included.

I. M. ROITT

1 · The active sites of immunoglobulin molecules

R. G. Q. LESLIE & S. COHEN *Department of Chemical Pathology, Guy's Hospital Medical School, London SE1 9RT*

I. Introduction

Specific combination of immunoglobulins (Ig) with the antigen which induced their synthesis constitutes the most characteristic feature of antibody molecules. This activity involves combining sites situated within the variable N-terminal sections of Ig molecules and its chemical basis has been extensively studied in recent years. The interaction of serum antibody and antigen has profound biological consequences concerned, for example, with the expression of acquired protective immunity and immediate hypersensitivity. There are, however, rather few instances in which the interaction of antigen with antibody leads directly to observable biological effects. Such primary reactions include the inactivation of enzymes and toxins [22] and the neutralization of some viruses [157, 148] and protozoa [25]. The biological expression of immune reactivity frequently requires secondary interactions of antigen-bound antibody with either the complement system or with specific cell surfaces. Such reactions involve specific sites which are located in the constant C-terminal sections of Ig molecules and may be activated only after combination of antibody with antigen. Current knowledge of the chemical structure and properties of the antigen binding and effector sites of Ig molecules is summarized below and possible mechanisms which mediate their functional interactions are discussed.

Antigen-binding sites of given specificity may occur on all classes of Ig whereas the effector sites are unequally distributed among classes and subclasses (Table 1.1). The biological consequences of immune reactions therefore depend fundamentally upon the relative class distribution of reacting antibodies. An ability to control and direct the class specificity of induced antibody synthesis is therefore an important practical goal of contemporary immunology. Induction of specific antibody synthesis is initiated by combination of antigenic determinants with B-cell surface receptors which appear structurally related to IgM [29, 131]. That is to say, among the class-specific C_H regions ($C\gamma$, $C\mu$, $C\alpha$, etc.) only $C\mu$, the heavy chain of IgM, appears to be synthesized independently of antigen stimulation during the course of ontogeny. Cγ (IgG heavy chain), which is not apparently represented in primitive cyclostome and elasmobranch fish, seems to be expressed only by cells which have previously synthesized Cμ. This underlies the IgM to IgG switch which occurs after antibody induction by many antigens [122, 172, 132]. Conversely, a failure of this switch may constitute the basis of low zone tolerance [173] and the defect of non-responder mice which produce IgM antibody normally during primary immunization, but fail to show an IgG response after secondary stimulation [65]. Whether the synthesis of all Cγ

Table 1.1. Properties of human immunoglobulins

	IgG	IgA	IgM	IgD	IgE
Structural					
Molecular weight	150,000	*160,000 (serum) 370,000 (secretory)	900,000	170,000	185,000
Heavy chains					
classes	γ	α	μ	δ	ϵ
subclasses	$\gamma_1\gamma_2\gamma_3\gamma_4$	$\alpha_1\alpha_2$			
percentage in serum	77, 11, 9, 3	90, 10			
Carbohydrate percentage	2·9	7·5	11·8	11·3	12·1
Biological					
Antibody activity	+	+	+	+	+
C fixation	+$\gamma_1\gamma_2\gamma_3$	0	+	0	0
Macrophage attachment	+γ_1 γ_3		+		0
Placental transfer	+γ_1 $\gamma_3\gamma_4$	0	0	0	0
Seromucous secretion	0	+$\alpha_1\alpha_2$	0	0	+
Tissue sensitization					
homologous spp.	0	0	0	0	+
heterologous spp.	−γ_1 $\gamma_3\gamma_4$	0	0	0	0†
Comb. staph. A. protein	+$\gamma_1\gamma_2$ γ_4	0	0	0	0

* Serum IgA is predominantly in the dimerized form in species other than human.
† Human IgE does sensitize monkey, but not guinea-pig tissues.

subclasses and of Cα, Cδ and Cϵ are antigen dependent and occur only in cells which have initially expressed Cμ has not been established. If this turns out to be the case, then the accumulation of IgA-producing cells beneath mucous surfaces must result from a Cμ to Cα switch occurring after antigenic stimulation and mediated by local influences active in these characteristic sites.

The possibility that humoral factors influence the class specificity of antibody is suggested by the Ig responses to certain infections. For example, helminth infections are associated with IgE antibody synthesis [123], visceral leishmaniasis with massive production of IgG and African trypanosomiasis with very high levels of IgM associated with both trypanocidal and other

IgM antibodies. These patterns of Ig production may have considerable significance because prolonged survival of obligate parasites indicates their capacity to evade the consequences of the host's immune reactions [24]. The investigation of such unusual Ig responses might conceivably identify mechanisms which influence the class specificity of antibody and so determine in part the biological consequences of immunization.

II. Basic structure of immunoglobulins

The 4-chain structure of Ig, consisting of 2 heavy and 2 light chains covalently linked by inter-chain disulphide bonds (Fig. 1.1) was originally proposed for

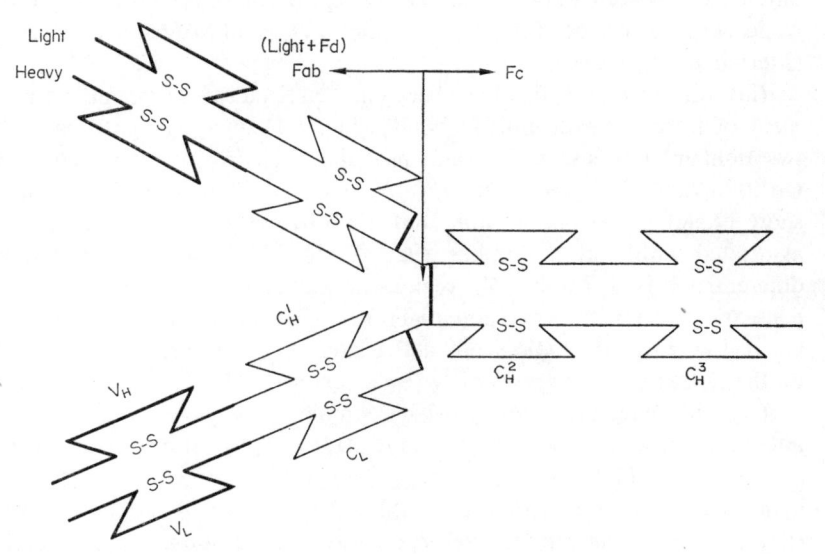

Fig. 1.1. Diagrammatic representation of the IgG molecule made up of 2 heavy and 2 light chains. Intra-chain disulphide bonds enclosing loops of 60–70 amino acids occur along the length of heavy and light chains. Heavy lines denote the N-terminal variable stretches of heavy (V_H) and light (V_L) chains. The arrow shows the site of papain digestion which splits within the hinge region of the heavy chain to give Fab and Fc fragments.

rabbit IgG [46], and is now known to apply to antibodies of all vertebrate species studied including primitive elasmobranch fish. The various classes and subclasses of Ig within a single species have common light chains and are differentiated on the basis of their heavy chains (reviewed by Cohen & Milstein [26]; Edelman & Gall [37]; Milstein & Pink [113]; Edelman [35]). High molecular weight antibodies such as serum IgM and sero-mucous IgA consist of covalently linked polymers of the 4-chain unit probably linked by a J-chain, which is rich in half-cysteine residues and common to both classes [116].

Certain general features of the basic Ig structure are of particular significance in regard to the location and properties of the active sites of antibody molecules.

(i) Ig chains contain an N-terminal variable region (V) comprising about 120 residues in which all heterogeneity within a subclass is localized. This was demonstrated first by Hilschmann & Craig [71] for human κ-chains, but V-regions of similar extent occur on all light and heavy chains.

(ii) The remaining C-terminal portions (C) of Ig chains within a given subclass have, by contrast, an invariant structure apart from differences attributable to allotypic specificity. The complete sequence of a human γ_1-chain has been elucidated [34] and considerable information is available for C-regions of other γ-subclasses [113], for the μ-chain [140] and, to a lesser extent, for the α-chain [59]. Available data reveal considerable sequence differences between heavy chain classes, e.g. between γ_1 and μ-chains [140] while subclasses show far greater homology, as illustrated by identity of C-terminal sequences.

(iii) All Ig chains which have been characterized show a periodic arrangement of intra-chain disulphide bonds (Fig. 1.1) dividing light chains into two domains (V_L and C_L), γ and probably α-chains into 4 domains (V_H, C_H^1, C_H^2 and C_H^3) and μ-chains into possibly 5 domains [49]. V_L and V_H show homology to one another but not obviously to C regions and are associated with antigen binding sites. V_κ and V_λ can be unambiguously differentiated [112, 72], but V_H regions appear common to all classes which consequently share the same potential range of antigen combining specificities. C_H regions carry the biologically active sites which are variously distributed on the classes and subclasses of Ig (e.g. human Igs, Table 1.1).

(iv) The heavy chain region which contains the Cys residues involved in interchain disulphide bonding shows considerable variation between classes and subclasses [49] and no homology with other sections of the heavy or light chain. This stretch of the γ- and α-chain is rich in proline and in all classes is highly susceptible to proteolysis. This section, on the basis of electron micrography and other physical measurements, has been designated the hinge-region (Fig. 1.1) since it permits free rotation of the Fab arms relative to Fc [44, 169].

(v) Mammalian species investigated in detail have several Ig classes which appear analogous to human IgG, IgA, IgM and IgE. In addition, the guinea-pig, mouse and rat have a homocytotropic antibody with no apparent counterpart in human serum. This is distinguished from IgE by resistance of homocytotropic properties to heating and sulphydryl reduction, relatively brief persistence at tissue sites of inoculation and high serum concentration after immunization. In the hamster [23] and rabbit [144] seemingly analogous 7S IgG$_1$ components do not have homocytotropic properties. This illustrates the extent of interspecies Ig variation and the difficulty of defining analogous classes and types in the basis of overall properties. Analogy can be established with certainty only by sequence data such as those which revealed that equine T-globulin, previously regarded as IgA on the basis of electrophoretic, antigenic and chemical properties, is a subclass of IgG [175].

III. Antibody-combining sites

(i) NATURE OF BINDING

Since antigen–antibody binding occurs in aqueous phase, the interaction of these reactants with water molecules plays an essential role in their specific combination. The main driving force towards complex formation arises from: (1) a decrease in enthalpy which accompanies substitution of bonding interactions between water and the antigen or antibody combining sites by more stable bonding interactions between antibody and antigen, (2) an increase in entropy primarily dependent on the release of bound water from the antibody and antigen active sites. This driving force, the unitary free energy of binding, has to overcome a decrease in entropy arising from the combination of two independent systems (antibody and antigen) into a single complex.

The relative contributions of different forms of non-covalent bonding in the antibody–antigen interaction are largely determined by the chemical nature of the solvent. The highly polar water molecules compete very effectively with antibody and antigen in H-bonding and ion-dipole interactions and so reduce considerably the contribution of these intrinsically strong forms of bonding, to the binding energy of complex formation. Ionic interactions may, however, be enhanced because charged groups in an environment of low dielectric constant, i.e. the antibody and antigen molecules, display increased ionic attraction relative to that between small oppositely charged molecules in aqueous solution. The limited data available suggest that ionic interactions may contribute only -1 to -2 kcal/mol [138], and H-bonding about -1 kcal/mol [130] to complexes for which the total free energy of formation lies in the range of -8 to -15 kcal/mol. London dispersion forces, which are dependent on the electronic polarizability of interacting groups, and are intrinsically weaker forces, are thought to make some contribution to binding, since the average polarizability of protein molecules is greater than that of water. However, a quantitative assessment of dispersion forces involved in the binding of benzoates, p-substituted with —CH$_3$, —Cl, —Br, —OCH$_3$, —NO$_2$, and —CH$_2$CONH$_2$ groups, has shown that the dispersion contribution, by substituents in this size range, may be less than -1 kcal/mol [130]. Little & Eisen [106], working with nitrophenyl haptens, proposed that electron transfer interactions between electron donating protein residues, e.g. tryptophan, and the electron accepting nitrated phenyl group, may play a part in complex formation. Estimation of the free energies of binding between di- and tri-nitrophenyl (DNP and TNP) amino caproates and free tryptophan (-0.65 and -1.5 kcal/mol, respectively) indicated that the contribution of electron transfer interaction amounted to only about 10 per cent of the net binding energy (-6 to -11 kcal/mol) of the immune complexes with these haptens. The binding contribution of permanent dipole–dipole interactions remain unexplored. It seems, therefore, that the contribution to binding by individual non-covalent interactions is small within a single hapten–antibody complex. However, these contributions are cumulative; for example, binding of the DNP Lys ligand by specific antibody may involve London dispersion forces, H-bonding and dipole interactions as well as electron transfer. The sum of these may amount to a substantial part of the total binding energy of complex formation.

The largest individual contributions to the free energy of binding arise from the coalescence of apolar, hydrophobic groups in an aqueous environment. The driving force does not arise from the weak interactions between the apolar surfaces (i.e. London dispersion forces), but from the increase in entropy which accompanies the release of water molecules from quasi-crystalline structures around apolar groups. This is illustrated by the observation that phenyl groups, in D-phenyl-(benzoyl amino) acetate, contribute $-4 \cdot 1$ kcal/mol to a total free energy of $-9 \cdot 1$ kcal/mol for binding with antibody [91]. This figure coincides with the free energy change for the transfer of 1 mol of benzene from an aqueous environment to liquid benzene [93]. An entropy contribution may also be important in ionic bonding where solvating water molecules are released on interaction of oppositely charged antigen and antibody sites.

The identity of amino acid residues involved in antigen binding by antibody has been explored, to a limited extent, by studying chemical modifications which alter specific antibody combination. The requirement of a complementary charge in the active site of antibodies against a charged hapten is demonstrated by the elimination of antibody activity against the cationic p-azo-phenyltrimethylammonium group which follows esterification of antibody carboxylate groups [61]. Similarly, involvement of argininyl and, to a lesser extent, lysyl side chains in anionic hapten binding has been demonstrated by modification of cationic groups in these residues [50, 57, 52, 63]. Iodination or acetylation of tyrosyl groups in antibodies specific for a variety of aromatic haptens sharply reduces antigen-binding activity [62, 64], but this observation does not necessarily localize the reactive residues within the combining site.

Although we have a general appreciation of the nature of antibody-binding activity, further analyses of individual antibody–antigen systems are essential for detailed understanding of the forces involved. Data, similar to those derived for substrate binding by the enzymes carboxypeptidase A [141], papain [8] or subtilisin BPN [143], where the orientation of the substrate within the active enzyme site and the individual binding interactions at specific subsites have been determined, are required to establish the chemical basis of antibody specificity. Such analyses are seriously complicated by heterogeneity of antibody structure and binding affinity which reflect chemical heterogeneity within active sites. Some progress has, however, been made in mapping the active sites of rabbit anti-poly-L-alanyl antibodies [151]. These bind the tripeptide, Ala_3, at three subsites, each of which binds a single alanyl group, but with quite distinctive affinities. The subsite which accommodates the amino-terminal alanyl residue binds with highest affinity and greatest specificity, while those binding the second and third residues show progressively weaker interactions; in addition, it was shown that the individual binding contributions are strictly additive.

(ii) ANTIBODY VALENCY

The existence of discrete antibody combining sites is indicated by competition for binding of cross-reacting haptens [99]. The studies of Pappenheimer *et al.* [128] indicated that there were two sites per 7S antibody and the subsequently established monovalency of Fab fragments [136] and symmetrical chain structure (H_2L_2) of IgG [47], were consistent with this. The valency of pentameric IgM ($H_{10}L_{10}$) has proved variable, but a recent study [33] using rabbit-anti-dextran and dextran determinants with molecular weights between 340 and 10^7 suggests that IgM has ten active sites but that binding of the larger antigens reduces the effective valency to five sites per antibody molecule.

Valency studies on two mouse myeloma IgA2 proteins with anti-dinitrophenyl activity [86, 167] have shown that the monomeric 7S forms of these immunoglobulins are divalent, consistent with their 4-chain structure. In the native state these proteins occur predominantly as 11S dimers, held together by a single J-chain, and are potentially tetravalent. A human IgA myeloma protein which binds nitrophenyl ligands was found to be tetravalent in its dimerized form [159]; whether steric restrictions, similar to those observed with IgM, reduce the effective valency of polymer IgA on combination with high molecular weight antigens is not known. The valency of IgE has not been determined directly. However, G and E antibodies from the same sera display comparable haemagglutinating activities [80] indicating that IgE is multivalent. Since IgE is composed of two heavy and two light chains, it is, presumably, divalent.

(iii) SIZE OF COMBINING SITES

The size of the antibody-combining sites has been assessed by determining the dimensions of antigenic determinants which give optimum binding (reviewed by Kabat [88]). Examination of the free energy of binding of isomaltose oligosaccharides by human anti-dextran antibodies, indicated that hexamers were bound optimally. Assuming that the sugar was bound in a fully extended form, this suggests that the combining site measures $34 \text{ Å} \times 17 \text{ Å} \times 6 \text{ Å}$ [88]. Similar studies employing oligopeptides [110, 91, 2] and large aromatic antigenic determinants lead to similar estimates and are consistent with the suggestion that 10 to 20 amino acids make contact with the antigenic determinant [92]. These estimates were made on sera taken after repeated immunization, which is characteristically associated with increasing antibody affinity and possibly with increasing size of combining sites. Evidence in favour of progressive enlargement of sites was obtained after immunization with a DNP-hapten attached to a defined sequence polymer [142] and with poly-L-aspartate bound to serum albumin [118]. However, Little & Counts [105] suggested that high affinity anti-DNP antibodies may have smaller combining sites than low affinity antibodies.

Electron microscopy of anti-DNP antibodies complexed with a divalent

DNP hapten [169] indicates that the binding site is situated at the extreme ends of the Fab regions. The length of the hydrocarbon backbone which links the two DNP groups indicates that the maximum depth of the site is about 10 Å. A similar estimate was obtained from ESR studies employing DNP haptens linked to a free radical by spacer chains of varying lengths [74]. When the distance between the hapten and the free radical was less than 10 Å, the latter was immobilized and an increased rotational correlation time for the free radical was observed.

(iv) ANTIBODY SPECIFICITY

The fact that antibodies react most strongly with the antigen which elicited their synthesis and show graded affinities for structurally related compounds is regarded as a basic immunological concept. The stereo-complementarity of the antigenic determinant and the antibody combining site is thought to provide the major contribution to specificity. Pauling & Pressman [130] attempted to correlate the affinities of related haptens with the degree of dilation required for their accommodation in a cavity defined by the antigenic determinant. A consistent relationship between these parameters indicated the importance of steric factors in combining specificity and suggested that the Van der Waal's contour of the hapten may approximate that of the antibody site to less than 1 Å.

Charged haptenic groups may contribute little to the binding energy between antigen and antibody [92], and yet play a determinant role in antibody specificity. Antibody produced against charged haptens displays reduced cross-reaction with uncharged analogues of almost identical configuration [138, 120]. The specific interaction of antibody with charged antigen is thought to involve neutralization of complimentary charges and the concomitant displacement of bound water molecules. Uncharged antigen analogues do not effectively displace bound water molecules, which consequently hinder access of the analogue to the active site. A similar effect may occur with antigenic determinants having groups capable of H-bond formation, since this can overcome the energy expenditure involved in displacement of water during combination of antigen with the antibody site. Appropriate orientation of hydrogen bonding groups may, therefore, play a part in antibody specificity.

Since stereocomplementarity is regarded as a major determinant of specificity, it is surprising that high affinity antibodies frequently show strong cross-reactions with related or even with quite distinct haptens. For example, anti-DNP antibodies with high affinity for the homologous antigen display greater cross-reactivity with the TNP analogue than do low affinity antibodies, and vice versa [107]. Antibodies selected for high affinity by fractional precipitation with the homologous ligand have virtually identical average intrinsic association constants for homologous and cross-reacting ligands. These observations suggest that whereas weak hydrophobic interactions between antigen and a closely fitting antibody site may be predominant in low affinity antibodies, additional stronger forces with less stereospecificity may operate in high affinity antibodies; their nature would presumably vary with the chemical identity of functional groups in the antigenic determinant.

A number of recent reports indicate that both induced antibodies [15, 89, 39] and individual monoclonal immunoglobulins [152, 39, 87] may bind two or more determinants having little or no structural relationship. This is illustrated by the reactivity of a single mouse monoclonal IgA protein (Table 1.2). Kabat et al. [89] suggested that cross-reactivity of anti-N purin-6-

Table 1.2. Reaction of mouse monoclonal IgA 315 with various ligands

Ligand	Association constant (litres per mole)
γ-DNP-aminobutyrate	7×10^7 [66]
DNP-β-alanine	$4 \cdot 9 \times 10^7$ [66]
ϵ-DNP-L-lysine	2×10^7 [66]
ϵ-DNP-D-lysine	$1 \cdot 7 \times 10^7$ [66]
δ-DNP-L-ornithine	$1 \cdot 4 \times 10^7$ [66]
2,4-dinitroaniline	9×10^5 [66]
α-DNP-L-leucine	$8 \cdot 7 \times 10^5$ [66]
Menadione	$6 \cdot 1 \times 10^5$ [39]
DNP-glycine	$2 \cdot 7 \times 10^5$ [66]
α-DNP-L-alanine	$1 \cdot 2 \times 10^5$ [66]
2,4-dinitronaphthol	$1 \cdot 1 \times 10^5$ [39]
Caffeine	$4 \cdot 6 \times 10^4$ [39]
5-Acetouracil caproate	$3 \cdot 2 \times 10^4$ [39]
Riboflavin	$2 \cdot 8 \times 10^4$ [39]
2,4-dinitrophenol	$\sim 4 \cdot 5 \times 10^3$ [66]

oyl antibodies with denatured DNA may depend largely on the arrangement of hydrophobic groups in the antigenic determinants. They demonstrated, using space filling models, that the homologous and cross-reacting ligands (N-purin-6-oyl glycine and 2'-deoxyadenylic acid, respectively) present a similar profile of hydrophobic centres when placed in appropriate orientations. Underdown & Eisen [166] reached a similar conclusion in their study of the interaction of 5 aceto-uracil amino caproate with high affinity rabbit and guinea-pig anti-DNP antibodies. A weak cross-reaction, only observed with a subset of the antibody population, is attributed to hydrophobic interactions, largely involving an aliphatic side chain, $(CH_2)_4$, common to both the immunogen (DNP-ϵ lysyl in the protein carrier) and the cross-reacting ligand. The greater cross-reaction of menadione with these antibodies and with mouse IgA_2 myeloma proteins displaying anti-DNP activity [39, 87] is attributed to the presence of electrophilic ring substituents which, as in nitrobenzenes, create positively charged aromatic nuclei that can form charge transfer complexes with electron donating residues in the antibody. In this connection, they note that certain enzymes also exhibit cross-reactions between naphthoquinones and DNP compounds, e.g. inhibition of a menadione reductase by 2.4 dinitrophenol [97].

Another explanation of unexpected cross-specificities arises from a study of the mouse myeloma IgA protein 460 which competitively binds 2.4 DNP-l-Lysine and 2-methyl 1.4 naphthoquinone thioglycollate (Men TG) [147]. Substitution of a single SH group, occurring in each combining region of protein 460, with DNP-S-S-DNP (10 Å, maximum dimension) diminishes Men TG binding but not DNP-l-Lys binding, while substitution with iodo-acetamide (3·5 Å, maximum dimension of the carboxymethyl group) affects neither. Papain digestion and denaturation with either 4·3M guanidium chloride or methyl sulphoxide causes selective alterations of one or other binding activity of protein 460. The authors conclude that the antibody cavity of protein 460 may contain more than one binding site and that DNP-l-Lys (18·2 × 7·9 × 3·9 Å) and Men TG (12·5 × 6·9 × 2·4 Å) might adhere to separate sites on opposite walls of the cavity, and that steric hindrance accounts for competitive inhibition of one ligand by the other.

The possibility that a single immunoglobulin may bind a number of chemically different antigens in different parts of the antibody cleft raises the question of how polyspecific immunoglobulins can give rise to antibody populations having a high degree of specificity towards a single hapten. Antigen induction of antibody synthesis involves binding to membrane receptors which are probably related to the antibody produced by the cell. If each antibody has several distinct specificities differently distributed in various molecular species, then it can be postulated that the dominant specificity of the antibody population will be that directed against the eliciting antigen and other specificities present in the combining regions will be diluted out [147]. The authors point out that this mechanism could also account for low levels of 'natural' antibodies commonly present in sera of animals not apparently exposed to the relevant hapten.

Certain observations are relevant to this interpretation of the data.

(a) Combining specificities identified on myeloma proteins may not be representative of induced antibodies of corresponding specificity. In the case of protein 460, the haptens tested are small in relation to the size of the combining sites which may possess higher affinity for another, larger determinant. In this connection, it is interesting that 2.4 dinitronaphthol is bound by protein 460 with an association constant twenty-fold greater than either of the haptens studied by Rosenstein and co-workers [87]. Further understanding of this problem may come from analysis of multiple combining specificities in homogeneous induced antibodies, such as those raised in rabbits against bacterial coat polysaccharides [38] or para-azo-benzoate [121, 146] or synthesized by cloned antibody cells proliferating either *in vivo* [3] or *in vitro* [96].

(b) Multiple specificities occur in normal antibody populations [39] and, as predicted, binding activities unrelated to the immunogen are confined to a minority subset of the total induced antibody. The anti-5-aceto-uracil activity of guinea-pig anti-DNP antibodies, for example, is restricted to 30 per cent of the anti-DNP population (cf. 96 per cent cross-reaction for the structurally related DNP/TNP system) [107].

(c) The hypothesis that antigen selects antibody having multiple potential binding sites is difficult to reconcile with the fact that high affinity rabbit anti-DNP and anti-TNP antibodies have distinctive tryptophan contents but virtually indistinguishable combining properties [107]. However, this particular difficulty applies equally to any antigen selection hypothesis, irrespective of whether unique or multiple binding activities are postulated for the specific site of a single antibody molecule.

(v) STRUCTURE AND LOCATION OF ANTIBODY COMBINING SITES

Direct evidence that antibody specificity is determined by amino acid sequence arose from a study by Buckley et al. [14]. Complete reduction and unfolding of Fab fragments produced concomitant loss of antibody activity and removal of the denaturant was associated with significant recovery of the original activity. This indicates that the chain folding which generates combining specificity is dependent on the primary sequence of the Fab fragments. The presence of variable sequences in human and mouse monoclonal proteins confined to the N-terminal portions of Fab fragments again suggested that primary sequences generate combining specificities. Analysis of the variable sequences that determine specificity has been hampered by the heterogeneity of most purified antibodies raised against even the simplest hapten and also by the rarity of myeloma proteins having specific binding affinities within the range for elicited antibodies. Such homogeneous antibodies [38] and monoclonal Igs with high combining affinity [40] do have uniform association constants and this confirms that primary sequences in V-regions determine both specificity and binding affinity.

Cathou & Werner [18] showed that the ORD and CD spectra of Fab fragments from anti-DNP antibodies, in varying concentrations of guanidium chloride, were stabilized by the presence of hapten. They concluded that the contact amino acids of the binding site were located in several non-consecutive portions of the polypeptide chain brought into close spatial relationship in the native conformation. A similar conclusion derives from comparative sequence studies on monoclonal proteins. Within the V-regions of both heavy and light chains, three short stretches with high sequence variability have been identified [177, 20, 94]. Two of these hypervariable stretches (at N26–34 and N89–98) are close to a Cys–Cys bridge, which occurs in all V-regions around N22 and N88. These data suggest that the hypervariable regions in both chains are brought into close proximity by disulphide bridging and appropriate folding to form the antibody cleft, and that specificity is determined by these hypervariable residues.

The precise location of combining sites has been sought by employing hapten determinants attached to a chemical group which will interact covalently with residues in or near to the active site. This technique of affinity labelling has the potential for providing direct information about the combining site, but has certain short-comings:

(a) If the active group is not an integral part of the antigenic determinant then interaction with adjacent, rather than contact, amino acids may occur. Such adjacent residues may, as a result of folding, be remote from the active site sequence.

(b) The identity of the reactive amino acid side chain is, in most cases, limited by the nature of the active group, e.g. diazo groups react only with tyrosyl, lysyl and histidinyl residues.

(c) In the case of induced antibodies, complexities may arise in identifying residues in regions of sequence heterogeneity.

Experiments which overcame most of these problems [56, 45, 67] provided results consistent with involvement of both light and heavy chains and, in particular, their hypervariable regions in the combining site. The importance of hypervariable regions is also indicated by the finding that of 10 mouse monoclonal λ-chains, 6 appear identical and 4 have amino acid substitutions confined to one or more of the 3 hypervariable stretches [174].

Conclusive evidence on the structure of the active site will be obtained most directly by X-ray crystallography of purified, homogeneous antibody fragments. Work in this direction progresses and the 6 Å resolution model of a crystallized Fab fragment from a myeloma protein has revealed a cleft of appropriate dimensions for an active site [135]. Better resolution of the crystal structure is required to identify the chain arrangement which leads to formation of the cleft. Kabat & Wu [90] postulated that nearest neighbour amino acids play an important role in determining the conformation of the middle amino acid so that angles of tripeptide sequences in the V-region of a κ-chain could be calculated from those in known proteins. In a 3-dimensional model of Vκ constructed on this basis, the two hypervariable regions, 23–34 and 89–97, form a pocket which could comprise part of the combining site, while the third hypervariable region occurs within a distance compatible with the estimated sizes of antigenic determinants.

IV. Ig effector sites

(i) LOCATION OF SITES

The IgG Fc fragment (molecular weight 50,000) prepared by papain hydrolysis (Fig. 1.2) retains many biological activities of the original molecule including the capacity to fix complement, attach to heterologous mast cells and B lymphocytes [129], combine with staphylococcal protein A, regulate IgG catabolic rate and cross the placental membrane and gut wall of the newborn (Table 1.3). The sites responsible for these properties are therefore contained within the two C-terminal intra-chain disulphide loops of the γ-chain (C_H^2 and C_H^3, Figs. 1.1 and 1.2). Smaller fragments of Fc, referred to as Fc′ or pFc′, which comprise only the C-terminal domain (C_H^3) can be prepared by hydrolysis with pepsin or papain (Fig. 1.2). These fragments carry some isotypic and allotypic determinants and combine with rheumatoid factors of certain specificities, but express no biological activities of the original Fc (Table 1.3). It is likely, therefore, that the N-terminal half of Fc (C_H^2, Fig. 1.2) contains many active sites characteristic of the γ-chain. Some evidence has been obtained for complement fixing activity in this region [95, 41] but the observed molar activities were equivalent to only about 5 per cent of that on the original Ig and are of uncertain significance. Some effector sites may be localized in the C-terminal C_H^3 domain, but lose their active configuration during enzymatic hydrolysis. This possibility is illustrated by

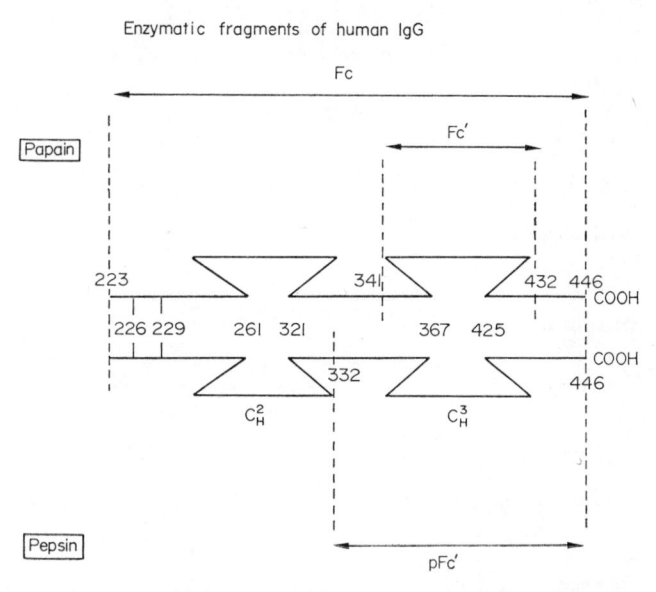

Fig. 1.2. Diagrammatic representation of the Fc fragment of human IgG$_1$ containing the C_H^2 and C_H^3 domains (Fig. 1.1) and showing sites of cleavage by papain and pepsin to yield Fc' and pFc' pieces containing the C_H^3 domain. Residues are numbered from the N-terminus; numbers in the centre refer to cystine residues (from [36, 164]).

the fact that both Fc' and pFc' contain the Gm(a) peptide, but only the latter, slightly larger, peptide expresses Gm(a) serological activity (Table 1.3).

Certain Ig effector sites appear to be localized in the F(ab')2 fragment, possibly within the C_H^1 domain (Fig. 1.1). Guinea-pig IgG$_1$ fails to fix complement in the presence of antigen or lyse antigen coated cells in the presence of complement. However, washed specific precipitates containing IgG$_1$ antibodies do fix complement [127] apparently beginning with C3. This sequence appears to be initiated when aggregated Ig activates a serum C3 proactivator to give a product with enzymatic action resembling C3 convertase [57]. The sites which fix C1q are present on the Fc fragment of IgG$_2$ but absent from IgG$_1$, whereas those which initiate the C3 shunt mechanism are present on F(ab')2 fragments from guinea-pig IgG₁ and IgG₂ [150] and probably also on human IgA [57]. Chan & Cebra [21] have provided evidence that the complement component, C4, may also attach preferentially to the Fab portion of Ig molecules, and there is some evidence for residual cytophilic activity in the F(ab')2 fragment of human IgG [75, 1]. It has also been suggested that stimulation of neutrophil leucocyte phagocytic activity by human and dog Ig fractions is retained by Fab but not by Fc [98].

Table 1.3. Properties of C-terminal regions of IgG. Data are for human IgG fragments except: * rabbit IgG fragments; † mouse IgG 2a

	Fc (C_H^2, C_H^3)	Fc' (C_H^3)	pFc' (C_H^3)	C_H^2
Synonyms			Component II Pep III	
Molecular weight	50,000 [136*]	21,000 [162] 24,000 [78]	26,000 [162] 25,000 [168]	
Isotypic specificity				
Class		+	+ [78]	
Subclass		+	− [78]	
Allotypic specificity				
Gm (a)		+	− [163, 78]	+ [70, 164] − [78]
Gm (non-a)		+	− [163]	+ [164]
Gm y		+		− [70]
Gm b¹		+	−	− [164]
Gm b⁰, b³, b⁴, b⁵		+	+ [163]	+ [164]
Biological activities				
Combination			− [78]	− [70]
Rheumatoid factor		+	+ [77, 165]	+ [165, 119]
Complement fixation		+	− [78, 165]	− [70, 165]	+ [95†]
Skin sensitization (heterologous)		+	− [78]	*− [137]
Membrane transmission placenta	+ [13*, 55]			
gut (new-born mouse)	*+ [115]		*− [137]	
Combination staph. A protein	+ [54]	− [54]	− [54]	
Control of catabolic rate	+ [43]	− [54]	− [54]	

Localization of biologically active sites in other classes of Ig has not been thoroughly studied. However, the Fc fragment of IgE which has a molecular weight of 94,000 contains the sites responsible for the attachment to isologous tissues [155] while its C-terminal Fc' fragment (molecular weight 57,000) is inactive in this regard [80]. The Fc fragment of human IgA has not been isolated, but mouse and rabbit IgA Fc can be prepared [42] and from the latter species binds the secretory component characteristically associated with seromucous IgA [100].

(ii) STRUCTURE OF Fc SITES

The failure to isolate active fragments from the Fc portions of Ig molecules has meant that the structure of the effector sites remains obscure. In addition, the remarkable diversity of activities associated with a given molecular species (e.g. IgG_1, Table 1.1), suggests that comparative sequence data are unlikely to identify those primary structures which generate sites mediating specific biological activities. The IgG sites which react with Clq and bind to macrophages and the IgE sites which attach to mast cells are all inactivated by mild reduction suggesting that integrity of inter-heavy chain disulphide bonds in the hinge region is essential [153, 1]. However, cleavage of this region with insoluble papain does not impair reactivity with complement [19]. Chemical modification of IgG by carbamylation or amidination of lysine or benzylation of tryptophane, substantially decreases complement binding and cytophilic activity without affecting antigen combining specificity or the ability to sensitize heterologous tissues for anaphylaxis [60, 111, 161].

Available evidence suggests that where the same biological activity is mediated by different Ig classes, the sites involved are structurally distinct. In some instances, the sites on different Ig classes appear to react with different receptors. For example, mouse 7S and 19S antibodies both bind to macrophages but not competitively, and only the 19S binding is dependent on the presence of Ca^{2+} ions [101]. In other instances, different Ig classes may bind the same receptor, but with significantly different affinities indicating that their reactive sites are structurally distinct. For example, measurement of the interaction of Clq with different classes of Ig by analytical ultracentrifugation, has shown that the affinity is greatest with IgG_3 and progressively less for IgG_1 and IgG_2 [117]. Similarly, both IgE and IgGa rat antibodies sensitize mast cells for histamine release, but the former has a higher affinity as indicated by long persistence at a site of injection and continued attachment to the mast cell surface after a washing procedure which readily elutes IgGa [170]. These two Ig classes compete for mast cell receptors so that pre-sensitization with IgGa, for example, can inhibit a subsequent IgE mediated reaction [6]. These findings indicate that the two Igs attach either to the same receptor by sites with different affinities or to distinct but closely adjacent receptors; in either case, the mast cell binding sites on the two Ig classes must be structurally different.

(iii) BINDING PROPERTIES OF SITES

Little direct information is available about the specificity of sites on the Fc section of Ig molecules. The class and subclass distribution of biological activities and instances of their separate inactivation by chemical treatment (see above) indicate that each is mediated but a separate specific site. The physicochemical nature of interactions between Fc sites and their receptors remain largely uncharacterized but reversibility indicates their non-covalent nature.

The Cl component of complement comprises three dissociable subunits of which Clq carries the binding site. This is a multichain protein of molecular weight of about 390,000 [179] comprising several subunits [158], and appearing to be pentavalent since it binds five molecules of IgG and one of IgM [117, 108].

(iv) CELL RECEPTORS FOR Fc SITES

Attempts to elucidate the nature of cell receptor sites for homocytotrophic and cytophilic antibodies have rested upon studying the effects of various enzyme and chemical treatments on the subsequent ability of receptor-bearing cells to react with the appropriate Ig or mediate the relevant biological response. This approach is limited by the fact that enzymes cannot be used which require a pH damaging to the cell under study, and also by the poorly defined specificity of many enzyme preparations which have been employed. Bach et al. [6], in carefully controlled investigations, studied the effect of 18 enzymes with defined specificities for protein, phospholipid and polysaccharide substrates, on the ability of rat peritoneal cells to sustain IgE-mediated reactions; their tentative conclusion was that the receptor contains sialic acid and the hydrophilic portion of membrane phospholipid. Alternative methods, such as the use of affinity chromatography, to isolate cell receptors which react with specific Ig classes have not been fully explored. Macrophages show a plateau of binding for ^{125}Ig which occurs at a level of about 2×10^6 sites per cell for rabbit IgG [133].

V. Initiation of Ig-mediated biological reactions

Several biological activities are mediated by sites which appear active on individual Ig molecules. This seems true of those which contribute to the control of Ig catabolic rate, mediate transfer across placental and gut membranes, and combination with staphylococcal protein A (Fig. 1.3a).

Catabolic mechanisms differ among classes of Ig since fractional breakdown rates of IgM and IgA are independent of serum concentration, IgD varies inversely with concentration [145], while IgG breakdown is concentration dependent in man and mouse. Fahey & Robinson [43] showed that the fractional rate of IgG catabolism was enhanced by infusion of either native IgG or the Fc fragment while Fab had no effect. Brambell et al. [12] suggested, on the basis of these findings, that native IgG molecules may bind to receptors by Fc sites and thereby be protected from catabolism and returned intact to the circulation, but no experimental evidence to substantiate this has been forthcoming.

Transmission of Ig from mother to foetus is a selective process occurring across the placenta in man and monkey and across the yolk sac splanchnopleure in the rabbit (reviewed by Waldmann & Strober [171]). In these species, IgG and its Fc fragment are readily transmitted, whereas Fab is not. In other species, antibody transfer occurs after birth across the gastro-intestinal tract. In ungulates this process seems to be non-specific and of brief duration but

(a) — Placental transfer
Gastro-intestinal transfer
Control catabolic rate
Combination staph aureus protein A

(b) — IgE mediated hypersensitivity

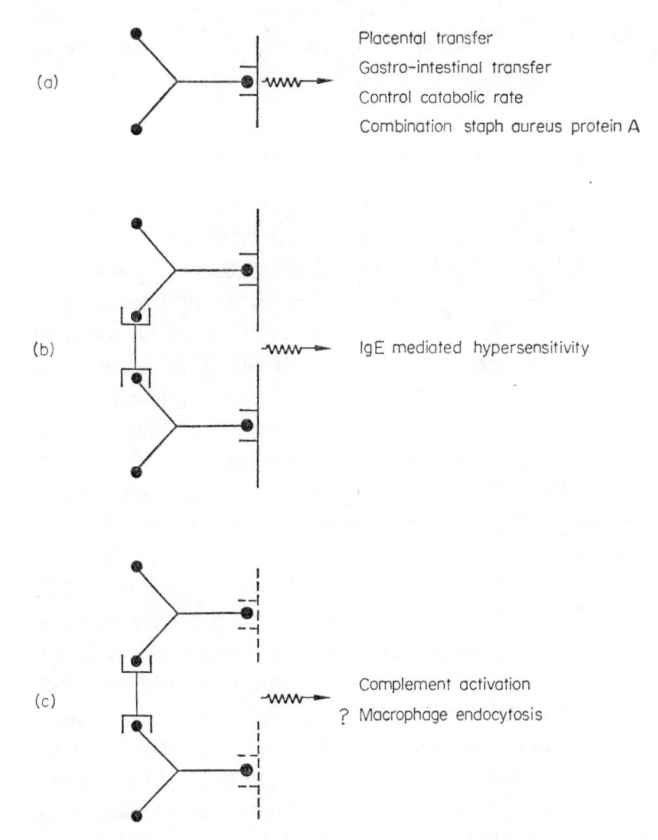

(c) — Complement activation
? Macrophage endocytosis

Fig. 1.3. Ig-mediated effector mechanisms. (a) Sites with biological activity in free antibody. (b) High affinity sites reactive on free antibody but requiring cross-linkage to trigger biological sequence. (c) Low affinity sites reactive on free antibody and requiring cross-linkage to trigger biological sequence.

in mice and rats transport is more prolonged (2–3 weeks) and is inhibited specifically by gastro-intestinal administration of IgG or its Fc fragment but not by Fab [114]. Specificity of transfer does not seem to involve selective uptake since pinocytosis occurs in microvilli of the placenta, yolk sac and newborn rodent gut. A selective attachment of IgG to specific receptors which facilitate transport across the cell was postulated by Brambell [11].

The protein A of *Staphylococcus aureus* combines with IgG molecules of several species and the active site is located on Fc [48]. This reaction may inhibit host defence mechanisms since protein A is anti-phagocytic for leucocytes in the presence of specific opsonins and bacteria [32] and presumably acts by binding to the Fc section of specific antibody and so blocking its opsonizing activity.

Several other reactions including immediate hypersensitivity, complement activation and possibly opsonization by macrophages, are not initiated by individual Ig molecules, but only by antibodies after combination with antigen (Fig. 1.3b, c). These reactions therefore require an antigen dependent interaction between Fab and Fc sections of Ig molecules and the nature of this has not been fully elucidated.

(i) CROSS-LINKING OF Ig IN THE INITIATION PROCESS

IgM and IgG antibodies in free solution combine reversibly with the first component of complement (Cl), but this does not initiate the subsequent steps of complement activation [117]. Hyslop et al. [76] who used guinea-pig complement and rabbit anti-DNP IgG antibodies in complexes with a divalent hapten found no complement binding with free antibody or with dimeric or trimeric antibody complexes. By contrast, large complexes involving four or more antibody molecules effectively fixed complement. This failure to demonstrate Cl fixation by monomeric Ig (see also Ishizaka et al. [81, 82]) may be due to different species or forms of Ig used.

In the case of antigen attached to cell surfaces, the interaction adjacent IgG molecules with Cl is sufficient to initiate the full cycle of lysis [10]. Antigen density on the cell surface is therefore a critical factor in determining the occurrence of complement mediated cytotoxic reactions [104]. For example, the failure of anti-Rh antibodies to fix complement is attributed to the comparative paucity of D antigen sites on the erythrocytic surface. Cohn [27] has suggested that the ability of IgG to mediate complement lysis in serum, but failure to initiate the same reaction in the Jerne plaque assay, can probably be attributed to the wide spacing of specific surface determinants which combine with the unique homogeneous antibody produced by a single cell. Similarly, the absorption of host components on to cell surfaces may alter the antigen density of established tumours and parasites, and permit their evasion of complement mediated cytolysis, which nevertheless remains effective against homologous cells newly introduced into the host—a phenomenon referred to as concomitant immunity [154].

Mast cells have homocytotropic antibodies (e.g. IgE) bound to their surface membranes, but are triggered for histamine release only after the bound molecules have become cross-linked usually by polyvalent antigen. By contrast, the majority of monovalent haptens are totally ineffective [102]. The requirement for cross-linking implies that the density of cell-bound IgE of given specificity is a critical factor determining antigen induced hypersensitivity. This is illustrated by the experiments of Prouvost-Danon & Binaghi [139] who showed that purified anti-DNP antibodies containing reagins effectively sensitized mouse cells in vitro whereas the original IgE-containing ascitic fluid from which the anti-DNP antibodies were purified, failed to specifically sensitize similar cell preparations. The nature of the cross-linkage between IgE molecules appears unimportant since multivalent antigen [102] and divalent anti-IgE antibodies [83, 85] are both potent initiators, whereas monovalent antigens or Fab fragments from anti-IgE antibodies are ineffective. Similarly, IgE chemically aggregated by bis-diazotization induces immediate hypersensitivity reactions in humans and guinea-pigs in the absence of other reactants, though the dosage required is about ten times that needed with immune complexes [84].

Studies on cytophilic antibody have shown that native Ig molecules of appropriate class bind to the surface of macrophages [9]; in addition, the attachment of antigen–antibody complexes to macrophages can be inhibited by excess free IgG [133]. These observations prove that cytophilic sites, at least on IgG, are available on the surface of native molecules. The studies of Phillips-Quagliata et al. [133] show that the amount of antibody bound to macrophages and the affinity of binding are increased by cross-linking with polyvalent antigen at equivalence, but are unaffected by monovalent or excess polyvalent antigen. Particles such as red blood cells, when reacted with cytophilic antibody, become attached to macrophages and remain bound to the surface if left at room temperature or 4°C. Incubation of such preparations at 37° causes phagocytosis of all attached red cells [9]. Phagocytosis occurs without complement when the opsonizing antibody is IgG [109] but the first four complement components are required for ingestion of membrane-bound particles coated with IgM [75]. Whether cross-linking of IgG by antigen is a required trigger for phagocytosis in unknown, since the influence of antigenic valency upon endocytosis has not been evaluated. The related process of pinocytosis (invagination of soluble material) can be stimulated directly by a macroglobulin present in bovine serum and having specificity for mouse erythrocytes and macrophages [28].

(ii) INITIATION MECHANISMS

There appear to be two ways in which cross-linking of antibody could initiate biological reactions which involve sites on Fc sections of Ig molecules.

(a) *Ig conformational change*

Combination with polyvalent antigen could expose or generate biologically active sites whose affinity is not fully expressed in the native molecule; combination with appropriate receptors would then trigger the biological event. This sequence would seem likely if native Ig did not bind receptors and did not inhibit binding by antigen–antibody complexes. In fact, as outlined above, the sites for Cl fixation, mast cell attachment and macrophage binding are all active in free homologous Ig of the appropriate class; it remains possible, however, that the binding affinity of Ig sites is increased or new sites are exposed by an antigen-dependent conformational change and that this triggers the receptor to initiate the biological sequence.

Such a conformational mechanism could, for example, explain the observed increase in binding affinity of cytophilic antibody after cross-linking by antigen. This hypothesis is also compatible with the demonstration that initial complement fixation associated with combination of anti-DNP antibodies with DNP conjugated red blood cells, is followed by an increase in C-binding affinity, within a multivalent domain, for subsequent C molecules [160]. This suggests that antibody in immune complexes may exist in two conformational states having a low free energy of transition, and that initial complement binding promotes a shift in the equilibrium towards the more active conformation. However, the existence of a similar equilibrium in the native antibody population is not excluded and nor is the possibility that the secondary binding is with bound complement which has itself undergone a conformational change after attachment to the antigen–antibody complex.

Physicochemical evidence for the postulated changes in antibody conformation after immune complex formation is scanty and available data are conflicting. Changes in optical rotation at a single wavelength observed when antibodies combine specifically with serum albumin, ferritin and a synthetic trivalent hapten [79, 69] indicate alterations in secondary or tertiary protein structure. Unambiguous assignment of conformational changes to the antibody cannot be justified when the antigen is also a protein contributing to the total optical rotation of the complex. Indeed, the evidence that larger protein antigens cause greater changes in optical rotation [69] might suggest that the antigen is an important contributor to the observed effects. ORD studies [156, 16, 18] reveal no change on complex formation of anti-DNP antibodies with monovalent antigen or with bivalent haptens [58] known to be effective in forming biologically active antibody complexes [76]. These findings led to the suggestion that the hinge region of antibodies may make no characteristic contribution to the ORD curve [58]. This seems likely as proteolysis of this region does not affect the ORD or circular dichroism of anti-DNP antibodies [156, 16] and nor does it affect the ORD of IgM [31].

Electron microscopy provides some evidence that combination with polyvalent antigens leads to opening of the Y-shaped antibody molecule with an increase in the angle between Fab arms [44, 169]. This could expose active sites in the hinge region, which are occluded in the native antibody molecule. Cathou and co-workers have estimated the inter-Fab angle (α) from the transient electric birefringence of IgG anti-DNP antibodies in solution [17] and have measured the minimum distance separating antigen combining sites in a hybrid anti-dansyl, anti-fluorescein antibody molecule by studying singlet–singlet energy transfer between the monovalent haptens [176]. They concluded that for immunoglobulins in solution, α invariably exceeds 80° and probably lies between 130 and 180°. A nanosecond emission anisotropy study of antibodies in solution supports the concept of a flexible molecule with each Fab section traversing an angular range of about 30° within nanoseconds [178]. Low angle X-ray scattering data on a human IgG$_1$ myeloma in solution [134] and the 6 Å resolution X-ray crystallographic study of Samra et al. [149] on another human myeloma IgG$_1$ are consistent with a T-shaped structure both in solution and in the crystal with α-invariant at 180°.

The results on immunoglobulins in solution therefore point to a flexible, open Y- or T-shaped IgG molecule, akin to electron micrographs of antibodies in multiple complexes with antigen. The closed conformation of free antibody, observed by electron microscopy may, it seems, represent a preparation artifact [176].

The finding that antibodies aggregated by many different chemical, physical and immunological means initiate similar biological activities has thrown doubt upon the idea that a specific conformational change is involved in these reactions. However, it is quite conceivable that different measures generate the same active site especially as human and rabbit IgG after heating, chemical denaturation, cross-linking or immune complex formation, carry new species-specific antigenic determinants irrespective of the method of aggregation [68].

(b) *Lattice formation*

The reactivity of effector sites on native Ig molecules and the failure to demonstrate convincingly antigen-mediated conformational changes in antibody molecules, leaves open the possibility that biological effects are induced by lattice formation which follows the interaction of Ig with multivalent antigen.

This could occur where the Fc regions of free antibodies have low affinity binding sites (e.g. for Clq or for macrophage receptors) so that antigen–antibody complexes have increased functional affinity by virtue of the number of sites in close proximity. In a multi-component system (such as the complement system) the increased functional affinity of the complex could cause retention of the first component for sufficient time to allow for activation and interaction with further components, thereby initiating the full sequence of the response. A similar mechanism seems possible for antibody-induced phagocytosis by macrophages.

The influence of multivalency upon overall affinity is illustrated by the fact that IgG antibodies have a functional affinity for antigen 10^3-fold greater and IgM antibodies 10^6-fold greater than the intrinsic affinity of their individual combining sites [73]. A similar correlation between functional activity and the number of reacting sites has been demonstrated in complement fixation. Thus, Augener et al. [4] have shown that free IgG and the 7S subunit of IgM bind similar amounts of Clq while pentameric IgM, which presumably contains 5 complement fixation sites per molecule, is 15 times more active. Larger aggregates of IgG and IgM bind up to 100 times more Clq on a weight basis. These data correlate with the observation that two or more IgG molecules in close proximity on the cell surface are required to produce a lytic lesion whereas a single IgM molecule is sufficient to produce the same effect [10].

The mechanism of mast cell degranulation mediated by IgE is of interest since the native antibody has a high affinity for cell surface receptors and yet stimulates histamine release only after cross-linking. The trigger may involve conformational changes within the antibody generating either additional binding activity or conformational changes within receptors at the cell surface. However, it is simpler to propose that lattice formation between bound IgE molecules leads to aggregation of cell surface receptors which provides a multivalent binding site for membrane or cytoplasmic components and alters membrane permeability in the locality of the aggregate. Mast cell degranulation requires activation of a serine esterase [7, 5], is inhibited by raised levels of cAMP [103, 84, 85, 124], is Ca and energy dependent in the final stage [103, 125] and is abolished by the action of cytochalasins A and B [126]. It seems probable that contractile microfilaments, activated by an influx of extracellular Ca^{2+}, play an important part in exocytosis of histamine containing granules [126]. Cyclic AMP may act either by controlling intracellular Ca^{2+} levels (cf. liver Ca^{2+} flux studies in rats [53]) or by modulating the activity of the serine esterase, possibly by phosphorylation of the enzyme (cf. inhibition by cAMP of glycogen synthetase through a phosphorylation step [30]). The latter proposal seems more probable since adenyl cyclase stimulators do not inhibit the last Ca^{2+} dependent stage of degranulation [103]. A role for the serine esterase has still to be described.

VI. Conclusions

Antibody molecules show a high degree of individual antigen-binding specificity and yet conserve certain biological properties, such as the capacity to fix complement, which characterize the class of Ig to which they belong. This functional dualism is generated by peptide chains which are unique in having variable N-terminal (V) regions and constant C-terminal (C-) regions.

The two antigen-binding sites of each 4-chain Ig molecule are contained within the V-regions of both heavy and light chains. Since specificity is determined by primary structure, it seems reasonable to conclude that combining sites within each chain comprise the two short hypervariable stretches brought into close proximity by an intra-chain disulphide bond, and a third hypervariable stretch presumably folded in the native molecule to within a distance compatible with the estimated size of antigenic determinants. The use of affinity labels has provided direct evidence that the hypervariable sequences of heavy and light chains actually constitute the antibody combining site. The stereochemical configuration of the antibody site is regarded as the prime determinant of specificity. It is therefore surprising that high affinity antibodies may show considerable cross-reactivity and may combine at high affinity with structurally unrelated haptens. This suggests that binding forces less dependent on stereochemistry can be predominant in such reactions; it is also possible that small haptens may interact with distinct or overlapping portions of relatively large, high affinity sites.

Biological effector sites occur predominantly in the Fc portion of the molecule which comprises the two C-terminal intra-chain disulphide loops of the heavy chains. There is virtually no information available about the detailed location, chemical structure, specificity or affinity of these sites. All appear accessible in native Ig and some, including those responsible for placental and gastrointestinal transfer of Ig molecules and the concentration dependent control of IgG catabolic rate, are active in free molecules. Other effector sites on free Ig molecules interact with their relevant receptors, but the full biological sequence is initiated only after the bound antibody has become cross-linked. This is true for complement activation, IgE-mediated hypersensitivity and possibly also for opsonin-induced phagocytosis.

The cross-linkage of Ig leads to lattice formation and may trigger the biological sequence by producing either aggregation or conformational change in the receptor. An Ig lattice signal is consistent with the known presence of effector sites on native Ig molecules, the failure of monovalent or excess polyvalent antigen to induce reactions and the triggering which occurs with diverse forms of cross-linking. Ig conformational changes may have a role in initiating biological reactions, but their occurrence does not seem mandatory.

References

[1] ABRAMSON N., GELFAND E.W., JANDL J.H. & ROSEN F.S. (1970) *J. exp. Med.* **132**, 1207.
[2] ARNON R., SELA M., YARON A. & SABER H.A. (1965) *Biochemistry* **4**, 948.
[3] ASKONAS B., WILLIAMSON A.R. & WRIGHT B.E. (1970) *Proc. natn. Acad. Sci. U.S.A.* **67**, 1398.
[4] AUGENER W., GREY H.M., COOPER N.R. & MULLER-EBERHARD H.J. (1971) *Immunochemistry* **8**, 1011.
[5] AUSTEN K.J. & BECKER E.L. (1966) *J. exp. Med.* **124**, 397.
[6] BACH M.K., BRASHLER J.R., BLOCH K.J. & AUSTEN K.F. (1971) In *Biochemistry o, the Acute Allergic Reactions*, eds. Austen K.F. & Becker E.L., p. 65. Blackwell, Oxford.
[7] BECKER E.L. & AUSTEN K.F. (1966) *J. exp. Med.* **124**, 379.
[8] BERGER A. & SCHECHTER I. (1970) *Phil. Trans. R. Soc. London, B* **257**, 249.
[9] BERKEN A. & BENACERRAF B. (1966) *J. exp. Med.* **123**, 119.
[10] BORSOS T. & RAPP H.J. (1965) *Science, N.Y.* **150**, 505.
[11] BRAMBELL F.W.R. (1966) *Lancet* ii, 1087.
[12] BRAMBELL F.W.R., HEMMINGS W.A. & MORRIS I.G. (1964) *Nature, Lond.* **203**, 1352.
[13] BRAMBELL F.W.R., HEMMINGS W.A., OAKLEY C.L. & PORTER R.R. (1960) *Proc. R. Soc. B.* **151**, 478.
[14] BUCKLEY C.E., WITNEY P.L. & TANFORD C. (1963) *Proc. natn. Acad. Sci., U.S.A.* **50**, 827.
[15] BUTLER V.P., JNR., BEISER S.M., ERLANGER B.F., TANENBAUM S.W., COHEN S. & BENNICH A. (1962) *Proc. natn. Acad. Sci., U.S.A.* **48**, 1597.
[16] CATHOU R.E., KULCZYCKI A. & HABER E. (1968) *Biochemistry* **7**, 3958.
[17] CATHOU R.E. & O'KONSKI C.T. (1970) *J. molec. Biol.* **48**, 125.
[18] CATHOU R.E. & WERNER T.C. (1970) *Biochemistry* **9**, 3149.
[19] CEBRA J.J. (1963) In *Conceptual Advances in Immunology and Oncology*, p. 220. Harper & Row, N.Y.
[20] CEBRA J.J., STEINER L.A. & PORTER R.R. (1968) *Biochem. J.* **107**, 79.
[21] CHAN P.C.Y. & CEBRA J.J. (1966) *Immunochemistry* **3**, 496.
[22] CINADER B. & LEPOW I.H. (1966) Antibodies to biologically active molecules. *Proc. 2nd Meeting Fed. Europ. Biochem. Socs.*, Vol. 1, p. 1. Pergamon Press, Oxford.
[23] COE J., PEEL L. & SMITH R.F. (1971) *J. Immun.* **107**, 76.
[24] COHEN S. (1973) *Clinical Aspects of Immunology*, eds. Gell P.G.H. & Coombs R.R.A., 3rd edition Blackwell, Oxford.
[25] COHEN S. & BUTCHER G.A. (1970) *Immunology* **19**, 369.

[26] COHEN S. & MILSTEIN C. (1967) *Adv. Immun.* **7**, 1.
[27] COHN M. (1971) In *Immunological Surveillance*, eds. Smith R.T. & Landy M. Academic Press, N.Y.
[28] COHN Z.A. & PARKS E. (1967) *J. exp. Med.* **125**, 1091.
[29] COOMBS R.R.A., FEINSTEIN A. & WILSON A.B. (1969) *Lancet* ii, 1157.
[30] DEWULF H. & HERS H.G. (1968). *European J. Biochem.* **6**, 558.
[31] DORRINGTON K.J. & TANFORD C. (1968) *J. biol. Chem.* **243**, 4745.
[32] DOSSETT J.H., KRONVALL G., WILLIAMS R.C. & QUIE P.G. (1969) *J. Immun.* **103**, 1405.
[33] EDBERG S.C., BRONSON P.M. & VAN OSS C.J. (1972) *Immunochemistry* **9**, 273.
[34] EDELMAN G.M. (1970) In *Developmental Aspects of Antibody Formation and Structure*, eds. Sterzl J. & Riha I., p. 381. Academia Publishing House, Prague.
[35] EDELMAN G.M. (1971) *Ann. N.Y. Acad. Sci.* **190**, 5.
[36] EDELMAN G.M., CUNNINGHAM B.A., GALL W.E., GOTTLIEB P.D., RUTISHAUSER U. & WAXDAL M.J. (1969) *Proc. natn. Acad. Sci., U.S.A.* **63**, 78.
[37] EDELMAN G.M. & GALL W.E. (1969) *A. Rev. Biochem.* **38**, 415.
[38] EICHMANN K., LACKLAND H., HOOD L. & KRAUSE R.M. (1970) *J. exp. Med.* **131**, 207.
[39] EISEN H.N., MICHAELIDES M.C., UNDERDOWN B.J., SCHULENBERG E.P. & SIMS E.S. (1970) *Fed. Proc.* **29**, 78.
[40] EISEN H.N., SIMS E.S. & POTTER M. (1969) *Biochemistry* **7**, 4127.
[41] ELLERSON J.R., YASMEEN D., PAINTER R.H. & DORRINGTON K.J. (1972) *FEBS Letters* **24**, 318.
[42] FAHEY J.L. (1963) *J. Immunol.* **90**, 576.
[43] FAHEY J.L. & ROBINSON A.G. (1963) *J. exp. Med.* **118**, 845.
[44] FEINSTEIN A. & ROWE A.J. (1965) *Nature* **205**, 147.
[45] FLEET G.W.J., KNOWLES J.R. & PORTER R.R. (1972) *Biochem. J.* **128**, 499.
[46] FLEISCHMAN J., PAIN R. & PORTER R.R. (1962) *Archs Biochim. Biophys. Suppl.* **1**, 174.
[47] FLEISCHMAN J., PORTER R.R. & PRESS E.M. (1963) *Biochem. J.* **88**, 220.
[48] FORSGREN A. & SJOQUIST J. (1967) *J. Immun.* **99**, 19.
[49] FRANGIONE B., PRELLI F., MIHAESCO C., WOLFENSTEIN C., MIHAESCO E. & FRANKLIN E.C. (1971) *Ann. N.Y. Acad. Sci.* **190**, 71.
[50] FREEDMAN M.H., GROSSBERG A.L. & PRESSMAN D. (1968a) *Biochemistry* **7**, 1941.
[51] FREEDMAN M.H., GROSSBERG A.L. & PRESSMAN D. (1968b) *Immunochemistry* **5**, 367.
[52] FREEDMAN M.H., GROSSBERG A.L. & PRESSMAN D. (1968c) *J. biol. Chem.* **243**, 6186.
[53] FRIEDMANN N. & PARK C.R. (1968) *Proc. natn. Acad. Sci. U.S.A.* **61**, 504.
[54] FROMMEL D. & HONG R. (1970) *Biochim. biophys. Acta* **200**, 113.
[55] GITLIN D., KUMATE J., URRUSTI J. & MORALES C. (1964) *Nature, Lond.* **203**, 86.
[56] GOETZL E.J. & METZGER H. (1970) *Biochemistry* **9**, 3862.
[57] GOTZE O. & MULLER-EBERHARD H.J. (1971) *J. exp. Med.* **134**, 90S.
[58] GREEN N.M. (1969) *Adv. Immun.* **11**, 1.
[59] GREY H.M., ABEL C.A. & ZIMMERMAN B. (1971) *Ann. N.Y. Acad. Sci.* **190**, 37.
[60] GRIFFIN D., TACHIBANA D.K., NELSON B. & ROSENBERG L.T. (1967) *Immunochemistry* **4**, 23.
[61] GROSSBERG A.L. & PRESSMAN D. (1960) *J. Am. chem. Soc.* **82**, 5478.
[62] GROSSBERG A.L. & PRESSMAN D. (1963) *Biochemistry* **2**, 90.
[63] GROSSBERG A.L. & PRESSMAN D. (1968) *Biochemistry* **7**, 272.
[64] GROSSBERG A.L., RADZINSKI G. & PRESSMAN D. (1962) *Biochemistry* **1**, 391.
[65] GRUMET F.C., MITCHELL G.F. & McDEVITT H.O. (1971) *Ann. N.Y. Acad. Sci.* **190**, 170.
[66] HAIMOVICH J., EISEN H.N. & GIVOL D. (1971) *Ann. N.Y. Acad. Sci.* **190**, 352.
[67] HAIMOVICH J., EISEN H.N., HURWITZ E. & GIVOL D. (1972) *Biochemistry* **11**, 2389.
[68] HENNEY C.S. & ISHIZAKA K. (1968) *J. Immun.* **100**, 718.
[69] HENNEY C.S. & STANWORTH D.R. (1966) *Nature, Lond.* **210**, 1071.
[70] HEIMER R. & SCHNOLL S.H. (1968) *J. Immun.* **100**, 321.

[71] HILSCHMANN N. & CRAIG L.C. (1965) *Proc. natn. Acad. Sci. U.S.A.* **53**, 1403.
[72] HOOD L. & EIN D. (1968) *Nature, Lond.* **220**, 764.
[73] HORNICK C.L. & KARUSH F. (1972) *Immunochemistry* **9**, 325.
[74] HSIA J.C. & PIETTE L.H. (1969) *Archs Biochem. Biophys.* **129**, 296.
[75] HUBER H., POLLEY M.J., LINSCOTT W., FUDENBERG H.H. & MULLER-EBERHARD H.J. (1968) *Science, N.Y.* **162**, 1281.
[76] HYSLOP N.E., DOURMASKIN R.R., GREEN N.M. & PORTER R.R. (1970) *J. exp. Med.* **131**, 783.
[77] IRIMAJIRI S., FRANGIONE B. & FRANKLIN E.C. (1966) *Arthritis Rheum. (N.Y.)* **9**, 860.
[78] IRIMAJIRI S., FRANKLIN E.C. & FRANGIONE B. (1968) *Immunochemistry* **5**, 383.
[79] ISHIZAKA K. & CAMPBELL D.H. (1959) *J. Immun.* **83**, 318.
[80] ISHIZAKA K. & ISHIZAKA T. (1971) *Ann. N.Y. Acad. Sci.* **190**, 443.
[81] ISHIZAKA K., ISHIZAKA T. & BANOVITZ J. (1965) *J. Immun.* **93**, 1001.
[82] ISHIZAKA K., ISHIZAKA T., SALMON S. & FUDENBERG H. (1967) *J. Immun.* **99**, 82.
[83] ISHIZAKA T., ISHIZAKA K., JOHANSSON S.G.O. & BENNICH H. (1969) *J. Immun.* **102**, 884.
[84] ISHIZAKA T., ISHIZAKA K., ORANGE R.P. & AUSTEN K.F. (1970) *Fed. Proc.* **29**, 575.
[85] ISHIZAKA T., ISHIZAKA K., ORANGE R.P. & AUSTEN K.F. (1971) *J. Immun.* **106**, 1267.
[86] JAFFE B.M., EISEN H.N., SIMMS E.S. & POTTER M. (1969) *J. Immun.* **103**, 872.
[87] JAFFE B.M., SIMMS E.S. & EISEN H.N. (1971) *Biochemistry* **10**, 1693.
[88] KABAT E.A. (1966) *J. Immun.* **97**, 1.
[89] KABAT E.A., BEISER S.M. & TANENBAUM S.W. (1966) *Cancer Res.* **26**, 459.
[90] KABAT E.A. & WU T.T. (1972) *Proc. natn. Acad. Sci. U.S.A.* **69**, 960.
[91] KARUSH F. (1956) *J. Am. chem. Soc.* **78**, 5519.
[92] KARUSH F. (1962) *Adv. Immun.* **2**, 1.
[93] KAUZMAN W. (1959) *Adv. Protein Chem.* **14**, 1.
[94] KEHOE J.M. & CAPRA J.D. (1971) *Proc. natn. Acad. Sci. U.S.A.* **68**, 2019.
[95] KEHOE J.M. & FOUGEREAU M. (1970) *Nature, Lond.* **224**, 1211.
[96] KLINMAN N.R. (1969) *Immunochemistry* **6**, 757.
[97] KOLI A.K., YEARBY C., SCOTT W. & DONALDSON K.O. (1969) *J. biol. Chem.* **244**, 621.
[98] LAHIRI A.K. & NAJJAR V.A. (1970) *Archs Biochem. Biophys.* **141**, 602.
[99] LANDSTEINER K. (1945) *The Specificity of Serological Reactions*, rev. ed. Harvard U.P., Cambridge, Mass.
[100] LAWTON A.R. (1970) Quoted by Gray, Abel & Zimmerman (1971) *Ann. N.Y. Acad. Sci.* **190**, 37.
[101] LAY W.H. & NUSSENZWEIG V. (1969) *J. Immun.* **102**, 1172.
[102] LEVINE B.B. (1965) *J. Immun.* **94**, 111.
[103] LICHTENSTEIN L.M. & BOURNE H.R. (1971) In *Biochemistry of the Acute Allergic Reactions, 2nd International Symposium*, eds Austen K.F. & Becker E.L., p. 161. Blackwell, Oxford.
[104] LINSCOTT W.D. (1970) *Nature, Lond.* **228**, 824.
[105] LITTLE J.R. & COUNTS R.B. (1969) *Biochemistry* **8**, 2729.
[106] LITTLE J.R. & EISEN H.N. (1967) *Biochemistry* **6**, 3119.
[107] LITTLE J.R. & EISEN H.N. (1969) *J. exp. Med.* **129**, 247.
[108] MACKENZIE M.R., CREEVY N. & HEH M. (1971) *J. Immun.* **106**, 65.
[109] MANTOVANI B., RABINOVITCH M. & NUSSENZWEIG V. (1972) *J. exp. Med.* **135**, 780.
[110] MAURER P.H. (1964) *Prog. Allergy* **8**, 1.
[111] MESSNER R.P., PARKER C.W. & WILLIAMS R.C. (1970) *J. Immun,* **104**, 238.
[112] MILSTEIN C. (1967) *Nature, Lond.* **216**, 330.
[113] MILSTEIN C. & PINK J.R.L. (1970) *Prog. Biophys.* **21**, 209.
[114] MORRIS I.G. (1963) *Proc. R. Soc. B.* **157**, 160.
[115] MORRIS I.G. (1964) *Proc. R. Soc. B.* **160**, 276.
[116] MORRISON S.L. & KOSHLAND M.E. (1972) *Proc. natn. Acad. Sci. U.S.A.* **69**, 124.
[117] MULLER-EBERHARD H.J. (1969) *A. Rev. Biochem.* **38**, 389.
[118] MURPHY P.D. & SAGE H.J. (1970) *J. Immun.* **105**, 460.

[119] NATVIG J.B. & TURNER M.W. (1970) *Nature, Lond.* **225**, 855.
[120] NISONOFF A. & PRESSMAN D. (1957) *J. Am. Chem. Soc.* **79**, 1616.
[121] NISONOFF A., ZAPPACOSTA S. & JUREZIZ R. (1967) *Cold Spring Harb. Symp. quant. Biol.* **32**, 89.
[122] NOSSAL G.J.V., WARNER N.L. & LEWIS H. (1971) *Cell Immun.* **2**, 41.
[123] OGILVIE B.M. (1964) *Nature, Lond.* **204**, 91.
[124] ORANGE R.P., AUSTEN W.G. & AUSTEN K.F. (1971a) *J. exp. Med.* (Suppl.). In *Symposium on Immune Complexes and Disease* **134**, 1365.
[125] ORANGE R.P., KALINER M.A. & AUSTEN K.F. (1971b) In *Biochemistry of the Acute Allergic Reactions, 2nd International Symposium*, eds. Austen K.F. & Becker E.L., p. 189. Blackwell, Oxford.
[126] ORR T.S.C., HALL D.E. & ALLISON A.C. (1972) *Nature, Lond.* **236**, 350.
[127] OSLER A.G., OLIVEIRA B., SHIN H.S. & SANDBERG A.L. (1969) *J. Immun.* **102**, 269.
[128] PAPPENHEIMER A.M., LUNDGREN H.P. & WILLIAMS J.W. (1940) *J. exp. Med.* **71**, 247.
[129] PARASKEVAS F., LEE S-T., ORR K.B. & ISRAELS L.G. (1972) *J. Immun.* **108**, 1319.
[130] PAULING L. & PRESSMAN D. (1945) *J. Am. chem. Soc.* **67**, 1003.
[131] PERNIS B., FORNI L. & AMANTE L. (1970) *J. exp. Med.* **132**, 1001.
[132] PERNIS B., FORNI L. & AMANTE L. (1972) *Ann. N.Y. Acad. Sci.* **190**, 420.
[133] PHILLIPS-QUAGLIATA J.M., LEVINE B.B., QUAGLIATA F. & UHR J.W. (1971) *J. exp. Med.* **133**, 589.
[134] PILZ I., PUCHWEIN G., KRATKY O., HERBST M., HAAGER O., GALL W.E. & EDELMAN G.M. (1970) *Biochemistry* **9**, 211.
[135] POLJAK R.J., AMZEL L.M., AVEY H.P., BECKA L.N. & NISONOFF A. (1972) *Nature New Biol.* **235**, 137.
[136] PORTER R.R. (1959) *Biochem. J.* **73**, 119.
[137] PRAHL J.W. (1967) *Biochem. J.* **104**, 647.
[138] PRESSMAN D. & SIEGEL M. (1953) *J. Am. chem. Soc.* **75**, 686.
[139] PROUVOST-DANON A. & BINAGHI R. (1970 *Nature, Lond.* **228**, 66.
[140] PUTNAM F.W., SHIMIZU A., PAUL C., SHINODA T. & KOHLER H. (1971) *Ann. N.Y. Acad. Sci.* **190**, 83.
[141] QUIOCHO F.A. & LIPSCOMB W.N. (1971) *Adv. Protein Chem.* **25**, 1.
[142] RICHARDS F.F., PINCUS J.H., BLOCH K.J., BARNES W.T. & HABER E. (1969) *Biochemistry* **8**, 1377.
[143] ROBERTUS J.D., ALDEN R.A., BIRKTOFT J.J., KRAUT J., POWERS J.C. & WILCOX P.E. (1972) *Biochemistry* **11**, 2439.
[144] RODKEY L.S. & FREEMAN M.J. (1969) *J. Immun.* **102**, 713.
[145] ROGENTINE G.N., ROWE D.S., BRADLEY J., WALDMAN T.A. & FAHEY J.L. (1966) *J. clin. Invest.* **45**, 1467.
[146] ROHOLT O.A., SEON B-K. & PRESSMAN D. (1970) *Immunochemistry* **7**, 329.
[147] ROSENSTEIN R.W., MUSSON R.A., ARMSTRONG Y.K., KONIGSBERG W.H. & RICHARDS F.F. (1972) *Proc. natn. Acad. Sci. U.S.A.* **69**, 877.
[148] ROSENSTEIN R.W., NISONOFF A. & UHR J.W. (1971) *J. exp. Med.* **134**, 1431.
[149] SAMRA V.R., SILVERTON E.W., DAVIES D.R. & TERRY W.D. (1971) *J. biol. Chem.* **246**, 3753.
[150] SANDBERG A.L., OLIVEIRA B. & OSLER A.G. (1971) *J. Immun.* **106**, 282.
[151] SCHECHTER I. (1970) *Nature, Lond.* **228**, 639.
[152] SCHUBERT D., JOBE A. & COHN M. (1968) *Nature, Lond.* **220**, 882.
[153] SCHUR P.H. & CHRISTIAN G.D. (1964) *J. exp. Med.* **120**, 531.
[154] SMITHERS S.R. (1972) *Br. med. Bull.* **28**, 49.
[155] STANWORTH D.R., HUMPHREY J.H., BENNICH H. & JOHANSSON S.G.O. (1968) *Lancet* ii, 17.
[156] STEINER L.A. & LOWEY S. (1966) *J. biol. Chem.* **241**, 231.
[157] STEMKE G.W. & LENNOX E.S. (1967) *J. Immun.* **98**, 94.
[158] SVEHAG S-E., MANHEM L. & BLOTH B. (1972) *Nature New Biol.* **238**, 117.
[159] TERRY W.D., ASHMAN R.F. & METZGER H. (1970) *Immunochemistry* **7**, 257.

[160] THOMPSON J.J. & HOFFMAN L.G. (1971) *Proc. natn. Acad. Sci. U.S.A.* **68**, 2730.
[161] THRASHER S. & COHEN S. (1971) *J. Immun.* **107**, 672.
[162] TURNER M.W. & BENNICH H.H. (1968) *Biochem. J.* **107**, 171.
[163] TURNER M.W., MARTENSSON L., NATVIG J.B. & BENNICH H.H. (1969a) *Nature, Lond.* **221**, 1166.
[164] TURNER M.W., NATVIG J.B. & BENNICH H.H. (1970) *FEBS Letters* **6**, 193.
[165] TURNER M.W., STANWORTH D.R., NORMANSELL D.E. & BENNICH H.H. (1969b) *Biochim. biophys. Acta* **188**, 265.
[166] UNDERDOWN B.J. & EISEN H.N. (1971) *J. Immun.* **106**, 1431.
[167] UNDERDOWN B.J., SIMMS E.S. & EISEN H.N. (1971) *Biochemistry* **10**, 4359.
[168] UTSUMI S. & KARUSH F. (1965) *Biochemistry* **4**, 1766.
[169] VALENTINE R.C. & GREEN N.M. (1967) *J. molec. Biol.* **27**, 615.
[170] VAZ N.M. & PROUVOST-DANON A. (1969) *Prog. Allergy* **13**, 111.
[171] WALDMANN T.A. & STROBER W. (1969) *Prog. Allergy* **13**, 1.
[172] WANG A.C., WILSON S.K., HOPPER J.E., FUDENBERG H.H. & NISONOFF A. (1970) *Proc. natn. Acad. Sci. U.S.A.* **66**, 337.
[173] WEBER G. & KOLSCH E. (1972) *Europ. J. Immun.* **2**, 191.
[174] WEIGERT M.G., CESARI I., YONKOVICH S.J. & COHN M. (1970) *Nature, Lond.* **228**, 1045.
[175] WEIR R.C. & PORTER R.R. (1966) *Biochem. J.* **100**, 63.
[176] WERNER T.C., BUNTING J.R. & CATHOU R.E. (1972) *Proc. natn. Acad. Sci. U.S.A.* **69**, 795.
[177] WU T.T. & KABAT E.A. (1970) *J. exp. Med.* **132**, 211.
[178] YGUERABIDE J., EPSTEIN H.F. & STRYER L. (1970) *J. molec. Biol.* **51**, 573.
[179] YONEMASU K. & STROUD R.M. (1971). *J. Immun.* **107**, 309.

2 · The cellular and molecular basis of immunological tolerance*

G. J. V. NOSSAL *The Walter and Eliza Hall Institute of Medical Research, Melbourne, Victoria 3050, Australia*

Immunological tolerance may be defined as that state, induced by the action of antigen, whereby the reactivity of a population of lymphocytes with respect to that antigen has been reduced or abolished. This definition gives emphasis to three aspects of non-reactivity, which distinguish tolerance from other states of diminished immunological responsiveness. First, tolerance is antigen-specific, in contrast to drug-induced, disease-associated or other generalized states of immunodepression. Secondly, tolerance is a property of the lymphocyte population, rather than of the animal as a whole; this sets it apart from, for example, antibody-mediated feedback inhibition of immunity. Thirdly, tolerance is caused by exposure of lymphocytes to antigen, and is thus different from reduced ability to respond to an antigen due to a peculiarity of immune regulatory or immunoglobulin structural genes. The best way of thinking of tolerance is as the exact opposite of immunological memory.

While this view of tolerance eliminates a proportion of cases of diminished responsiveness to antigen, it is a mistake to think that all the phenomena covered by the term tolerance must have an identical and unique causal mechanism. Many of the confusing paradoxes in the current literature on tolerance disappear if one admits that the same end result can be achieved in widely differing ways. The challenge then remains of determining which of the many elaborate experimental models of tolerance best approximates to 'true' tolerance, i.e. the non-reactivity we display to our own blood and tissue antigens. Here, too, it is becoming clear that we must be at least a little pluralistic, and admit of at least two, and probably more, ways in which self-tolerance is achieved.

As it is not the purpose of the present group of essays to present a comprehensive review, it will be necessary to begin with a set of postulates about the immune response to provide a backdrop for an analysis of tolerance. Much documentation of the experiments which justify these postulates in the field of immunity [1–4] and tolerance [5–8] is provided in recent reviews. The

* This is Publication No. 1784 from the Walter and Eliza Hall Institute.

more controversial extensions of the postulates will be taken up later in this essay.

KEY CONCEPTS OF CELLULAR IMMUNOLOGY RELEVANT TO MECHANISMS OF ANTIGEN ACTION

1   Adaptive immune responses involve the activation of lymphocytes by antigen. In most, if not all, circumstances this activation involves cell proliferation and the generation of specific effector cells.

2   Lymphocytes involved in immunity belong to two distinct families, called T and B lymphocytes for short. T lymphocytes arise in the thymus, and are seeded out from there into the secondary lymphoid organs such as lymph nodes and spleen. When activated by antigen, T lymphocytes and their progeny subserve the phenomena of cell-mediated immunity. These include the type of inflammatory response known as delayed hypersensitivity, the destruction of allografts, the graft-versus-host reaction and the non-complement-dependent killing of tumours. T lymphocytes are also of importance in helping B lymphocytes to respond to antigen, and in most *in vivo* situations, antibody formation is abnormal in animals lacking T cells. Many T lymphocyte functions involve other cells as the final mediators of the immune phenomenon. B lymphocytes arise from the same multipotent stem cells, resident chiefly in the bone marrow, as do T lymphocytes. Their differentiation is independent of the thymus. In birds, it takes place in a thymus-like organ known as the bursa of Fabricius, but in mammals, stem cells differentiate into B cells by mechanisms and in sites that are still unknown. After activation, B lymphocytes and their progeny synthesize large quantities of antibody, and are thus essential for humoral immunity.

3   Activation of lymphocytes depends on interactions between determinant groups on antigen molecules and specific receptor molecules at the lymphocyte surface. These receptors are membrane proteins. In the case of B cells, the receptors are clearly immunoglobulin molecules. In the case of T cells, the nature of the receptors is more controversial, some workers supporting the view that the receptors are also immunoglobulins, and others stating that a different, as yet chemically undefined, series of recognition molecules is involved.

4   The physico-chemical basis of interaction between lymphocyte receptor and antigenic determinant differs fundamentally from that of other macromolecular recognition systems such as enzyme-substrate interactions or DNA–RNA hybridization, in that great variation in affinity of binding is a key hallmark of the system. It is evident that one receptor molecule can bind many antigenic determinants, though with varying binding strength. Similarly one antigenic determinant can interact with many diverse receptors. The recognition system is degenerate and redundant, a situation which

confers advantages when the receptors do not 'know' what antigens they will encounter [9].

5 A given lymphocyte, in both the B [10, 11] and T [12, 13] series, displays a very restricted sample of the full range of receptors which the whole animal possesses. It is not known whether each lymphocyte displays only *one* kind of combining site or recognition unit on its surface, though it *is* known that one antibody-forming cell secretes a unique, monomolecular species of antibody molecule. *see Nature 250: 669-71*

6 In both T and B cell series, the receptors displayed on the lymphocyte surface prior to antigen exposure reflect the immune response capacity of the cell. If cells capable of binding a given antigen are removed from a population, the lymphocytes which remain respond less well or not at all to that antigen [10–13]. Unpublished evidence is slowly coming forward to show the converse, namely that cell populations enriched for lymphocytes with receptors for a given antigen respond to that antigen with greater strength than does the starting population.

7 The simplest view of lymphocyte activation, and one consistent with all the facts, is that Burnet's clonal selection theory [14] is correct for both T and B cells. In other words, a lymphocyte has only one molecular species of antibody displayed on its surface. The events of activation result in the increased production of that unique serologic specificity, subject only to the qualification that a clone may switch the kind of heavy chain constant region which it chooses to attach to the combining sites of the secretory product [15]. The question of whether clonal selection is *strictly* correct, or whether a virgin lymphocyte displays a restricted small *set* of receptors, still representing only a tiny fraction of the whole universe of immunoglobulins, is unlikely to be resolved experimentally during the currency of this book. Therefore, for the rest of this essay, I will adopt the *one cell–one receptor* position as the simplest and the most appealing to me. This position needs special justification for the T cell, which will be given below.

8 The molecular basis of antigenic signalling to lymphocytes is unknown. However, it is known that some agents can mimic the effects of antigen, in causing blast transformation, cell division and synthesis of specialized proteins by lymphocytes. An early event following the attachment of some of these agents to the lymphocyte surface is a spatial re-arrangement of membrane receptors. Thus, bivalent antiglobulin antibodies cause the Ig receptors of B lymphocytes to cluster into patches (by a cell metabolism independent process), and then to form a 'cap' over one segment of the cell (through a metabolism-dependent process) [16, 17]. Monovalent Fab fragments of antiglobulins do not cause this change, nor do they cause blast transformation of lymphocytes. Receptor re-arrangement can be inhibited by a variety of means, and theories of cell signalling, based on induction or failure of re-arrangement, are being discussed [18].

9 Clonal selection is not to be thought of as the result of a single encounter between a single receptor and a single antigenic determinant at a single point in time. There is good evidence to show that clones of antibody-forming cells can vary greatly in size, depending on antigen dose and efficacy, or otherwise, on negative feedback mechanisms. At the level of a single responsive cell, it is clear that receptor molecules turn over metabolically [19, 20]; that capping can be followed by extensive receptor regeneration [21] and re-capping [22]; and that antigen-induced signals can be reversed by trypsinization of the antigen-binding lymphocyte [23]. This implies that any molecular model of immunity-tolerance signal discrimination must have a time dimension as well as a space dimension.

10 The T cell helper effect in antibody formation is not a marginal phenomenon or a laboratory artefact, but a major factor in the control of the immune response. Some B cells can be triggered by direct interaction between a repeating series of identical antigenic determinants and surface Ig receptors. This is particularly the case for responses confined to IgM antibody production [24, 25]. Most *in vivo* responses, and particularly those involving the IgG or IgA classes of antibody, require T cell help [26, 27].

TWO MECHANISMS BY WHICH T CELLS MAY HELP ANTIBODY PRODUCTION

If the T helper effect is crucial to immunity, it must be discussed before tolerance can be analysed. A key to understanding this phenomenon is the fact that most antigen molecules possess more than one region of their surface that constitutes an antigenic determinant. It turns out that a T cell response against one portion of an antigenic mosaic helps the B cell response towards another portion. The most clear-cut experiments in this field have been done using hapten-protein conjugates as antigens, and measuring the amount of antibody formation against the hapten [28, 29]. Let us term the hapten H and the carrier protein C. Then, anti-H B cells can be triggered by the antigen HC only when anti-C T cells are simultaneously activated. This T cell activation can be achieved by using either HC or C as antigen. If anti-C T cells are activated, but an antigen HD is used in an attempt to get anti-H antibody production, the end result is usually only slightly more anti-H antibody than in the absence of any T cell activation. In other words, collaboration does not work well unless T cells are responding to the particular carrier to which the hapten of the stimulating antigen is attached. Some exceptions to this rule have been found [2]. For example, if a very vigorous T cell response is produced, a non-specific augmentation of many B cell responses may ensue. This suggests the existence of a specific and a non-specific influence of T cells on B cell function.

Tissue culture experiments, though capable of being models for only part of the complex series of events leading to *in vivo* immune responses, lend themselves well to an analysis of T–B collaboration. Experiments by Feldmann, Marchalonis and colleagues [30–34] have led us to adopt the following working hypothesis, more fully explained elsewhere [32], which is summarized under the next three subheadings.

T CELL RECEPTORS

We believe that T cells recognize antigens by means of surface immunoglobulin receptor molecules, the chemical nature of which is very similar to the 7S IgM on the surface of B cells. We base this claim on the fact that direct chemical study of the T cell surface by a radiochemical method [33, 34] has demonstrated IgM-like (or IgT) molecules on T cells, and has shown that the binding specificity of these receptors mirrors the immunological specificity of the T cell population. Further, T cell reactions to antigens, be these stimulatory [35] or inhibitory [13] can be blocked by pretreating the T cell with antiglobulin antibody. We are aware of certain failures to repeat this finding [36] and of the fact that antiglobulins do not 'see' the T cell receptor as readily as the B cell receptor [37]. We cannot yet clarify the circumstances, possibly related to receptor embedding or anchoring in the membrane, which are at the root of this difference. This is certainly an important area for future research. The second big argument against the T cell receptor being Ig is that it does not explain either (a) the genetic linkage between T cell response capacity and immune regulatory genes situated in the H2 region [38]; or (b) the high degree of reactivity of T cells to allogeneic histocompatibility antigens [12, 39]. The former, but not the latter, finding would be explained if an IgT structural gene were situated between the H2-d and the H2-k ends of the H2 region [40]. The third objection to the concept of an Ig family of molecules as T cell recognition units relates to the apparently broader cross-reactivity of T cell responses, and the absence of helper effects between two haptens linked to a single carrier. This suggests that T cell receptors recognize a *broader area* of a molecule than do Ig molecules. I believe that most immunologists overestimate the specificity of Ig. It may be that as many as 1 or 2 per cent of all immunoglobulins can bind specifically to a given antigenic determinant [9–80]. If this is so, most of the findings regarding T cell specificity could be explained using the concept of a lower median triggering threshold in T cells than in B cells. Operationally, the ready activation of cells with low-affinity receptors (each receptor recognizing a molecular structure of the size of three to five amino acids as for IgG) might be difficult to distinguish from effects resulting from a recognition system based on molecules with a wider or deeper area of macromolecular complementarity. On balance, I am at the present more impressed with the positive evidence for T cell IgT receptors than with the negative arguments, and it is reassuring to note that the subject is being so intensively investigated that definitive experimental resolution of the problem should only be two or three years away.

NON-SPECIFIC PRODUCTS OF T CELL ACTIVATION

T cells are activated by antigen, through mechanisms that are not yet understood but may involve macrophages [41, 42] and even T–T collaboration. Blast transformation, clonal division and production of effector T cells with antigen specificity ensues [43]. During this activation process, the T cells secrete a group of highly potent, immunologically non-specific substances known as lymphokines. It appears that one, at least, of these substances is capable of increasing the response of B cells to antigens, under circumstances where those B cells are making a detectable but suboptimal response to antigen [44, 45, 46, 30, 31]. The chemical nature of this B cell-stimulatory material is not known, but it is clear that it can boost the B cell response to any antigen, even T cell-independent ones. Arguments have been put forward to imply that this is the chief, or possibly even the sole, way in which T cell activation helps B cell responses [2]. The apparent need for a chemical linkage between the hapten triggering the B cell and the carrier triggering the T cell in many cell collaboration models could then be explained by postulating that the factor or inducer made by T cells had a very short biological half life or range of action. On that view, only B cells held near to T cells by an antigen bridge effect would get the help required. Such a short range of action seems incompatible with the rather robust character of the stimulatory agent in tissue culture systems whose environment mimics much of the *milieu interieur* of lymphatic tissues. I am convinced of the validity of the non-specific factor, but prefer to consider it as a relatively minor one in most physiological immune responses.

SPECIFIC PRODUCTS OF T CELL ACTIVATION [30–34]

On our view, T cells also produce an immunologically specific helper factor. This, we believe, is the IgM-like molecule, identical to its receptor, which may be termed IgT. IgT differs from 7S IgM in having a marked tendency to become associated with macrophage-like cells (Cone, Feldmann, Marchalonis & Nossal, unpublished results). Strong evidence exists that IgT, complexed to antigen, can attach to macrophages, and that such macrophages can be washed and can stimulate B cells in the absence of further antigen. If the IgT is anti-C, the H portion of the antigen HC would be left free at the macrophage surface and could react with anti-H receptors on B cells.

This mechanism serves to concentrate antigen at a particular point, namely the macrophage membrane, allowing the possibility of multi-point binding of antigenic determinants to B cells, which may be essential to B cell receptor re-arrangement and triggering. It is also possible that the macrophage may play some active stimulatory role in helping B cells. It is certainly intriguing to see that, during the early proliferative phase of an immune response, some lymphocytes spend a considerable period closely attached to the macrophage surface, and frequently divide while still in intimate contact with the dendritic macrophage [47].

The postulate of a third cell as an essential element in T–B collaboration preserves the concept of 'antigen-focusing' [48] as the chief function of helper T cells, but removes the requirement that two *rare* cells (the anti-C T cell and the anti-H B cell) must meet. The great tendency for IgT to adhere to macrophages may explain why IgT is not found in the serum. Finally, there is no need to postulate large scale secretion of IgT. A gentle metabolic turnover of surface receptors would suffice for the focusing function.

KEY EXPERIMENTAL RESULTS OF THE T AND B LYMPHOCYTE ERA RELEVANT TO TOLERANCE MECHANISMS

Most of the large body of data on the phenomenon of immunological tolerance was accumulated before the crucial role of T cells in humoral immune responses was appreciated. It has thus become necessary both to repeat many old experiments but using defined lymphocyte populations, and to reinterpret old data in the light of the new facts. From this exciting period, the following concepts seem the most relevant to theories of tolerance [1–8].

1 As regards immunological tolerance induced experimentally to foreign antigens, it is much easier to achieve tolerance in T than in B cells [49–52]. T cell tolerance requires a lower antigen dose and less time; it lasts longer, and can be induced with many antigens, even those that do not persist well in extracellular fluids. B cell tolerance has been unequivocally demonstrated in only a few systems. In models using monomeric protein antigens, tolerance can be induced only following large doses of antigens with prolonged extracellular half-lives, and even in such cases, only affects B cells with high affinity for the antigen. B cell tolerance in model systems employing polymeric antigens with multiple repeating determinants will be discussed separately below.

2 If an animal has been exposed to a tolerance regime which has successfully rendered the T cells tolerant, but has left the B cell population normally reactive, this animal will behave as if tolerant. In other words, when the tolerizing antigen is injected in an immunogenic form, e.g. as an aggregate, the animal makes a grossly suboptimal response, particularly if the IgG response is measured. However, if the antigen in question, or certain determinants on it, are injected coupled to another carrier protein, an immune response ensures. This is because a different (non-tolerant) T cell population is activated by the new carrier, and can help the B cells (which are themselves normally reactive) to respond.

3 As regards the tolerance that we possess to the proteins and carbohydrates of our own body, it is probable that we have both T and B cell tolerance to those 'self' antigens present in high concentration in extracellular fluid. For many self antigens which reach the blood stream in only low concentrations, we may possess only T cell tolerance. It is not necessary to postulate that either B or T cell tolerance to self antigens must be complete. Low levels of antibody to various self antigens can be present in health just as low levels of antibody to foreign antigens can occur in animals that are nevertheless profoundly tolerant. If, however, a self antigenic determinant to which there is T cell, but not B cell, tolerance is introduced coupled to a non-tolerated carrier, extensive antibody formation can occur through the mechanisms described above, and disease can result [53]. It may be that agents which are great non-specific stimulants of T cells, such as Freund's complete adjuvant, can cause the release of so much B-cell stimulating factor as to encourage T-cell independent antibody formation under some circumstances. This may be one mechanism at work in some of the laboratory models of auto-immune disease.

4   Soluble complexes of antigen and antibody can have a profound tolerance-inducing effect on lymphocytes [4, 6, 54]. So far the effect has been best worked out for B cells, but there are reasons to believe that it can work for T cells also. There are many circumstances where sensitive methods exist to test for the antibody component of such complexes but not for the antigen. Under such circumstances, the phenomenon may masquerade as enhancement. I believe that many enhancement phenomena, particularly those involving passive transfer of small amounts of serum rest on a *central* mechanism of this type, involving tolerance induction by antigen–antibody complexes. It is also possible that the blocking factors which are present in the serum of some cancer patients, and which can inhibit the *in vitro* cytotoxic killing of tumour cells by the patients' own lymphocytes, are soluble antigen–antibody complexes [55]. The ways in which such complexes block the function of lymphocytes may not obey all the criteria of tolerance, but much more work needs to be done on the relationships between blocking factors, enhancing antibodies and antibody-mediated tolerance.

5   Some forms of experimentally induced tolerance are rapidly reversible when the antigen source is withdrawn [56–58]. Not all of these models have been fully analysed in terms of T and B cell tolerance. Similarly, cells which have attached to their surface an *excess* of a stimulatory lectin, and which do therefore not commence DNA synthesis, can be caused to do so if the excess lectin is removed and the cell is exposed to a stimulatory lectin concentration [59]. *In vitro* tolerance induction of B cells by polymerized flagellin can, during the first 16 h of incubation, be reversed by trypsinizing bound antigen off the B cell surface [23]. There is little doubt, therefore, that circumstances can be found in which a cell considered to be tolerant can be induced to become reactive again. The question is whether tolerance induction, as it occurs physiologically towards self antigens, involves such reversible mechanisms. This question cannot be resolved experimentally at present. Mechanisms may exist to eliminate *in vivo* the cells with high avidity receptors for self determinants.

IN VITRO INDUCTION OF TOLERANCE

A widely held view of tolerance has been that monomeric proteins reaching the lymphocyte surface tend to induce tolerance, whereas macrophage-associated [60] or T-cell associated [61] antigen tends to cause immune induction. In many *in vivo* situations, de-aggregated antigens do act as tolerogens whereas aggregated or particulate antigens are immunogenic [62]. If this simple view were correct, it should be possible to induce tolerance readily *in vitro* with soluble, monomeric antigens. In fact, this turns out to be difficult and, in many cases, apparently impossible. *In vitro* tolerance induction in both T and B cells has been intensively investigated in my laboratory over the last five years [4, 32, 54, 63, 64]. Cells are held for 6 to 24 h under tissue culture conditions with the putative tolerogen, and are then washed and either re-incubated under conditions ideal for an *in vitro* response, or injected adoptively into an irradiated host. Under such circumstances, B cells can be rendered tolerant with relatively low (but still supra-immunogenic) concentrations of antigen, but only if the tolerogen exhibits many repeating units of the same antigen on a single molecular aggregate. Considerably lower (and now sub-immunogenic) concentrations of antigen can tolerize when soluble antigen–antibody complexes are used in the zone of antigen excess. However, soluble monomeric protein antigens cannot tolerize B cells *in vitro* even when the highest practicable molar concentrations are used. Close spacing of antigenic determinants on a carrier can favour tolerance, and distant spacing can favour immunity [64]. Our study of T cell tolerance induction *in vitro* is much less advanced (J.W.Schrader & M.Feldmann, in preparation). Helper T cells are harvested from carrier-primed mice, and the cell population is then tested for its capacity to help B cells mount an anti-hapten response. Induction of tolerance is tested by pre-incubating the T cells with various concentrations of carrier protein, either in monomeric form or attached to a polymerized particle, creating a carrier matrix with repeated determinants. Tolerance in this setting means inhibition of the helper effect. It turns out that soluble, monomeric protein *can* achieve such tolerance while unable to tolerize B cells. This is consistent with the *in vivo* conclusion that T cells are easier to tolerize than B cells. However, much lower concentrations of carrier achieve the same effect if the tolerogen is attached to polymerized particles. The question of antibody-mediated induction of T cell tolerance remains to be studied in detail.

RELEVANCE OF *IN VITRO* MODELS TO *IN VIVO* REALITIES

The various *in vitro* tolerance models from our own and other [21, 65] laboratories present us with somewhat of a dilemma when contrasted with the bulk of *in vivo* tolerance work. In fact, the model tolerogens are often good immunogens *in vivo*, and the best *in vivo* tolerogens act poorly *in vitro*. Logically, there are only two ways out of this situation: either the *in vitro* models represent some sort of artefact not relevant to *in vivo* tolerance mechanisms; or else, the demonstrated *in vitro* mechanisms do not work *in vivo* because of some complexity not present in tissue culture. Let us examine each alternative in turn.

The question of whether the *in vitro* tolerance is an artefact is perhaps best illuminated by considering the elegant series of experiments on *in vivo* tolerance induction conducted by Howard and his colleagues using polymeric polysaccharide antigens [66–70]. With the type-specific carbohydrate of *Diplococcus pneumoniae* known as S III, an antigen which produces a good, thymus independent immune response in low dose, a prolonged state of specific tolerance can be produced in the B lymphocyte population by a single injection of a relatively high dose. This tolerance is preceded by a small amount of antibody formation; is of long duration in the animal, associated, in all probability with prolonged persistence of the poorly digestible antigen; but is readily lost when the cells are transplanted into an antigen-free environment. The *in vivo* tolerance induced by ourselves to *Salmonella* polymerized flagellin shares some features with this model [71]. It is possible that a population of 'reversibly tolerized' B cells exists in such animals, analogous, perhaps, to the B cells studied *in vitro* [23] which have absorbed sufficient polymerized flagellin on to their surface to become tolerant, but which can be 'rescued', at least for a certain period of time, by trypsinization to remove the tolerogen from the lymphocyte surface. The other antigen studied by Howard's group, polyfructose or levan, is also a thymus-independent antigen. Tolerance to this carbohydrate is *not* preceded by immunization, is also long-lasting, and is not reversed when cells are exposed to an antigen-free environment. This tolerant state looks like the result of the specific removal of reactive B cells, recovery being dependent on repopulation from stem cells. It may have some features in common with the irreversible *in vitro* tolerance to polymerized flagellin which occurs when the tolerogen has been present for three days, and which is not reversible by trypsin [23].

Another more general but equally important argument to show that *in vitro* tolerance studies have *in vivo* relevance is in the analysis of enhancement. Quantitative considerations show that most enhancement procedures *cannot* work through a covering-up of antigenic sites on the target tumour or grafted tissue. A central mechanism implicating inhibited lymphocytes is more likely. It now becomes imperative to analyse *in vitro* antibody mediated tolerance with T cells as targets. The success obtained with multi-determinant tolerogens suggests that this may work well.

Let us now look at the second possibility, namely that *in vivo* conditions differ greatly from *in vitro* ones. This needs examination for both polymeric and monomeric molecules. Antigens like polymerized flagellin certainly are removed very rapidly from extracellular fluid by the large reservoir of phagocytic cells present *in vivo*. Their half-life in the circulation is measured in minutes. This would militate against tolerance induction by the *in vitro* mechanism unless frequent multiple injections were given. In fact, it is possible to achieve tolerance to such antigens *in vivo* using daily injection protocols. The carbohydrate antigens which give good *in vivo* tolerance after a single injection may do so by virtue of being stored inside macrophages, followed by gradual, prolonged release.

What of *in vivo* conditions and monomeric protein antigens? Three possibilities for the differential effects *in vivo* and *in vitro*, particularly on the B cell population, suggest themselves. First, the process of tolerogenesis by monomers (whatever it is) may take several days, and tissue culture of mouse lymphocytes is not yet sufficiently advanced to keep non-stimulated cells in a physiological state for that length of time. Secondly, monomers may not tolerize as monomers *in vivo*; rather, they may be converted into soluble antigen–antibody complexes through union with natural antibody, in other words they may tolerize by the powerful antibody-mediated tolerance mechanism. Thirdly, the *in vitro* model may lack some element vital for tolerogenesis. This may be macrophages to phagocytose the antigen-coated cell [70], some necessary micro-environmental factor, or a third possibility that we must now consider in detail.

TOLERANCE AS A RESPONSE OF IMMATURE T OR B CELLS?

Both T and B cells possess receptors for antigen but come from stem cells which lack such receptors. Could it be that differentiating T and B cells go through a transient phase, perhaps just after the receptors first appear at the surface, during which any contact with antigen is a signal for cell death [72]? If so, cells with receptors for self antigens would be 'nipped in the bud', as it were, perhaps transiently appearing at their site of origin [73] but never reaching the peripheral lymphoid organs in significant numbers. Antigens entering from the outside might also tolerize a few cells (if they reached the thymus or bursa equivalent, which they may not) but would be rapidly eliminated through the activation of the more differentiated competent cells. Such a mechanism would harness the fact that self antigens are always present, but foreign antigens are pulsed in unexpectedly. This mechanism remains entirely speculative but retains some attractions. Of course, it includes an element lacking in the *in vitro* models, as *in vitro* tolerance tests effects on differentiated and not differentiating T and B cells. If such a mechanism were the sole one operating, one could make certain predictions about the kinetics of tolerance induction. If a monomeric, non-immunogenic protein were introduced, it could produce no effect on the mature B and T cells already competent in the secondary lymphoid organ, but could stop new cells of this type being generated. The tolerance induction rate would then parallel the rate of spontaneous death of competent T and B cells. We know that some T and B cells are long-lived, but these may represent mainly cells that have already contacted antigen. We have little information about the life span of *virgin* cells freshly seeded out from the primary lymphoid organs. However, on balance it is probably fair to say that in some systems [5, 49, 70, 74] tolerance induction is too rapid to be plausibly explained by the above as the sole mechanism. It is possible, however, that the mechanism *does* operate but is supplemented by one or more 'fail safe' mechanisms, such as antibody-mediated tolerance, to cope with cells that 'slip through' the tolerance-sensitive differentiation phase.

INFECTIOUS TOLERANCE AND THE ROLE OF IgT

In most experiments in the tolerance field, the assumption is made that tolerance is essentially a negative quality or an absence of reactivity from a cell population. Recently, the challenging concept of infectious tolerance has been put forward [75]. Tolerant cells are added to normal cells and the mixed population is tolerant. On this view, T cells of tolerant animals are seen as manufacturing something that actively suppresses response capacity of B cells. The mechanism of infectious tolerance has not yet been worked out, but it is clear that the phenomenon is not universal; it is far more common for a mixture of tolerant and normal cells to behave as normal rather than as tolerant. One explanation of infectious tolerance (Feldmann, unpublished) would fit in well with the concept of T–B collaboration presented above. If T cells were stimulated excessively, an over-production of IgT might result. This could functionally saturate macrophages, and allow complexes of IgT and antigen to reach the lymphocyte surface directly. This could lead to tolerance of antibody-mediated type, similar to that induced by IgG–antigen complexes.

ANTIGEN-BINDING CELLS IN TOLERANT ANIMALS

Much controversy rages around the question of whether 'tolerant cells' exist, i.e. cells with receptors for a given antigen, that have been reversibly shut off by that antigen, but which, as the antigen disappears, revert to immune competence. Some aspects of this subject have been covered already. At first glance, an easy test of the question might be to count the number of cells able to bind radioactively labelled antigen present in the lymphoid tissues of animals at various stages of tolerogenesis. If tolerance implies a killing of cells, such antigen-binding cells (ABC) should progressively disappear. Unfortunately, this approach turns out to have certain complexities. First, ABC as usually measured [76] consist mainly, if not solely, of B lymphocytes. Secondly, tolerance in the B cell compartment may only affect the high affinity B cells [51], leaving low affinity cells unaffected, or possibly even increased in number, thus leading to paradoxical ABC counts. Thirdly, it is not clear whether a 'tolerant cell' would or would not have enough of its surface sites unoccupied by antigen to give a positive reaction in the ABC test. Thus, it is no wonder that investigators in this field have produced results which vary from no change, decrease or even an increase in the observed ABC counts [74, 77–79]. Perhaps the most convincing results in this field come from studies in which the response capacity of the B cell population is directly monitored as a kinetic function of time after administration of the tolerogen [74]. This shows close parallelism between falling response capacity and falling ABC numbers. While this is consistent with clonal elimination as the tolerance mechanism, it is equally consistent with *in vivo* receptor saturation. I have already indicated that reversibly tolerant cells exist in certain experimental circumstances. Whether reversibly tolerant, long-lived, self-antigen-coated lymphocytes are the norm *in vivo* is another question. It is not illogical to suppose that nature may have devised some mechanism for eliminating such useless and perhaps dangerous entities, but definitive experiments are lacking.

FUTURE APPROACHES TO TOLERANCE MECHANISMS

As organ transplantation, auto-immune diseases and non-rejection of antigenic cancers remain important clinical problems, there will, no doubt continue to be a large amount of experimental work performed on tolerance, enhancement and blocking phenomena involving *in vivo* studies and chemically poorly defined antigens. Nevertheless, it is likely that the central molecular and cell biological mechanisms involved in tolerance will only be solved using precise *in vitro* approaches.

Much more remains to be done using lectins and antiglobulins as models. These agents can trigger lymphocytes, and pretreatments that interfere with this triggering [18, 59] may help elucidate the basis of tolerance. While the model substances have the advantage of triggering most or all lymphocytes of a particular type, they have the disadvantage that none accurately mimics an antigen in its mode of triggering. Even antiglobulins do not unite with the antibody combining site of the receptor as do antigens, but with the Fc part. This could produce grossly different allosteric effects on the receptor molecule. Therefore, it is predictable that workers will progressively switch to cell populations which have been enriched for lymphocytes with a particular antigen-binding capacity [80], and will study the effects of real antigens, capable of triggering a substantial percentage of the cells.

What parameters of cell function will be measured? It is clear the the phenomenon of patch and cap formation [16, 17] represents a real breakthrough and raises many issues for study with antigens rather than antiglobulins. Antigens do cause capping [21, 80], and it may be that we will learn much about tolerance by defining the conditions of antigen molarity, molecular arrangement, and duration of presence in the tissue culture medium which are required for an inhibition of such capping. Also, we need to know how antigen affects the inherent metabolism of Ig receptors. These are spontaneously shed and regenerated in normal lymphocytes [19, 20]. After a cycle of capping and regeneration, they may be present at the cell surface in increased amount [21]. What happens if antigen is continuously present for hours or days? Can repeated cycles lead to over-stimulation and cell death? Can monomeric antigen affect the cell in any way other than to block the subsequent triggering by bivalent or multivalent antigen? Do cells cap or fail to cap with tolerogenic antigen–antibody complexes?

Receptor re-arrangement is one window into the events at the cellular level, but others exist. With cell populations enriched for ABC, it should be possible to correlate effects outlined above with parameters such as adenyl cyclase levels, and RNA and DNA synthetic rates. Ideally, these in turn should correlate with the final generation of progeny effector cells, either forming antibody or mediating cellular immunity. In such an ideal model system, one could study the effects of antigen dose and form first on receptor flow, then on cell metabolism and finally on clonal expansion; and each study could be performed separately for T and B cells. Similarly, the model could be used to probe the various effects of agents that have been said to lower lymphocyte triggering thresholds, such as products of T cell activation, poly-adenylic:poly-uridylic acid and factors from activated macrophages.

Another need for the future is to devise tissue culture systems for the *in vitro* genesis of new T and B cells from stem cell precursors. It seems unlikely that the idea of a tolerance-sensitive phase in the lymphocyte's differentiation will be resolved any other way. Anything that can be revealed about the effects of antigen on cells with newly formed receptors would be helpful.

Two real difficulties exist in the scenario for tolerance research outlined above. The first is a simple logistic one. Will any group of investigators be willing or able to apply all the relevant methodologies to a single model system so that it can be studied from all these perspectives? So far, the tolerance field has suffered from a plethora of models, and there has been great difficulty in extrapolating from one to the other. Secondly, no matter how excellent the tissue culture model, it will never fully reflect the complexities of the *in vivo* situation. Any insights which the reductionist approach may generate will have to be critically evaluated in *in vivo* tolerance experiments, messy as these may be.

The reader will, by now, have gathered that the title of my essay has promised too much. We do not know the molecular and cellular mechanisms behind tolerance. We do, however, have many new tools to aid us in our search. The black box where antigen enters on one side, and immune cells exit out the other seems a little less impenetrable. Even the brief 'tolerance is dead' phase, which followed over-enthusiastic reaction to the realization of the importance of enhancing antibodies, has been laid to rest by Brent *et al.* [81], allowing an honoured place for both classical tolerance and blocking factors. Real progress has been made since the experimental birthday of this field [82], forming a sturdy springboard for future adventures.

References

[1] NOSSAL G.J.V. & ADA G.L. (1971) *Antigens, Lymphoid Cells and the Immune Response.* Academic Press, New York and London.
[2] KATZ D.H. & BENACERRAF B. (1972) *Adv. Immun.* **15**, 1.
[3] MILLER J.F.A.P. (1972) *Int. Rev. Cytol.* **33**, 77.
[4] FELDMANN M. & NOSSAL G.J.V. (1972) *Q. Rev. Biol.* **47**, 269.
[5] WEIGLE W.O. (1973) *Adv. Immun.* **16**, in press.
[6] MÖLLER G. (ed.) (1972) *Transplant. Rev.* **8**, 3–136.

[7] BRENT, L. (1971) In *Immunological Tolerance to Tissue Antigens*, ed. Nisbet N.W. & Elves, M.W., p. 49. Orthopaedic Hospital, Oswestry, England.
[8] DRESSER D.W. & MITCHISON N.A. (1968) *Adv. Immun.* **8**, 129.
[9] EDELMAN G.M. & GALLY J. (1973) *Adv. Genet.* in press.
[10] ADA G.L. & BYRT P. (1969) *Nature, Lond.* **222**, 1291.
[11] WIGZELL H. (1970) *Transplant. Rev.* **5**, 76.
[12] FORD W.L. (1971) *Nature New Biol.* **234**, 178.
[13] BASTEN A., MILLER J.F.A.P., WARNER N.L. & PYE J. (1971) *Nature, Lond.* **231**, 104.
[14] BURNET F.M. (1957) *Aust. J. Sci.* **20**, 67.
[15] NOSSAL G.J.V., WARNER N.L. & LEWIS H. (1971) *Cellular Immun.* **2**, 41.
[16] TAYLOR R.B., DUFFUS W.P.H., RAFF M. & DE PETRIS S. (1971) *Nature New Biol.* **233**, 225.
[17] LOOR F., FORNI L. & PERNIS B. (1972) *Europ. J. Immun.* **2**, 203.
[18] YAHARA I. & EDELMAN G.M. (1972) *Proc. natn. Acad. Sci. U.S.A.* **69**, 608.
[19] WILSON J.D., NOSSAL G.J.V. & LEWIS H. (1972) *Europ. J. Immun.* **2**, 225.
[20] MARCHALONIS J.J., CONE R.E. & ATWELL J.L. (1972) *J. exp. Med.* **135**, 956.
[21] DIENER E. and colleagues (1972) *Proc. nat. Acad. Sci. U.S.A.* **69**, 2364.
[22] PERNIS B. (1972) Personal communication.
[23] DIENER E. & FELDMANN M. (1972) *Transplant. Rev.* **8**, 76.
[24] FELDMANN M. (1972) *Europ. J. Immun.* **2**, 130.
[25] HOWARD J.G. (1972) *Transplant. Rev.* **8**, 50.
[26] BANKHURST A. & WARNER N.L. (1972) *Aust. J. exp. Biol.* **50**, 661.
[27] CREWTHER P. & WARNER N.L. *Aust. J. exp. Biol.* **50**, 625.
[28] MITCHISON N.A. (1971) *Europ. J. Immun.* **1**, 68.
[29] FELDMANN M. & BASTEN A. (1972) *Europ. J. Immun.* **2**, 213.
[30] FELDMANN M. & BASTEN A. (1972) *J. exp. Med.* **136**, 49.
[31] FELDMANN M. (1972) *J. exp. Med.* **136**, 737.
[32] FELDMANN M. & NOSSAL G.J.V. (1973) *Transplant. Rev.* **13**, 3
[33] MARCHALONIS J.J., CONE R.E., ATWELL J.L. & ROLLEY R.T. (1973) In *The Biochemistry of Gene Activation in Higher Organisms*, ed. Lee J.K. & Pollack J.L., in press.
[34] CONE R.E., SPRENT J. & MARCHALONIS J.J. (1972) *Proc. natn. Acad. Sci. U.S.A.* **69**, 2556.
[35] WARNER N.L. (1971) In *Contemporary Topics in Immunobiology*, p. 1. Plenum Publishing Corp., New York.
[36] CRONE M., KOCH C. & SIMONSEN M. (1972) *Transplant. Rev.* **10**, 36.
[37] RAFF M.D., STERNBERG M. & TAYLOR R.B. (1970) *Nature, Lond.* **225**, 553.
[38] MCDEVITT H.O. & BENACERRAF B. (1969) *Adv. Immun.* **11**, 31.
[39] JERNE N.K. (1971) *Europ. J. Immun.* **1**, 1.
[40] COHN M. (1973) In *The Biochemistry of Gene Expression in Higher Organisms*, ed. Lee J.K. & Pollack J.L. Aust. and N.Z. Publishing Co., Sydney, in press.
[41] LONAI P. & FELDMAN M. (1971) *Immunology* **21**, 867.
[42] WAGNER H., FELDMANN M., SCHRADER J.W. & BOYLE W. (1972) *J. exp. Med.* **136**, 331.
[43] SPRENT J. & MILLER J.F.A.P. (1972) *Cellular Immun.* **3**, 385.
[44] SCHIMPL A. & WECKER E. (1971) *Europ. J. Immun.* **1**, 304.
[45] KATZ D.H., GOIDL E.A., PAUL W.E. & BENACERRAF B. (1971) *J. exp. Med.* **133**, 169.
[46] DUTTON R.W., FALKOFF R., HIRST J.A., HOFFMAN M., KAPPER J.W., KETTMAN J.R., LESLEY J.F. & VANN D. (1972) In *Progress in Immunology*, ed. Amos B., p. 355. Academic Press, New York.
[47] MATTHES M.L., AX W. & FISCHER H. (1971) *Z. ges. exp. Med.* **154**, 253.
[48] MITCHISON N.A., RAJEWSKY K. & TAYLOR R. (1970) In *Developmental Aspects of Antibody Formation and Structure*, ed. Sterzl J., p. 547. Publ. House Czech. Acad. Sci.
[49] WEIGLE W.O., CHILLER J.M. & HABICHT G.S. (1972) *Transplant. Rev.* **8**, 3.

[50] MITCHISON N.A. (1971) In *Cell Interactions and Receptor Antibodies in Immune Responses*, ed. Mäkelä O., Cross A. & Kosunen T., p. 249. Academic Press, New York and London.
[51] RAJEWSKY K. (1971) *Proc. R. Soc.* (B) **176**, 385.
[52] MILLER J.F.A.P. & MITCHELL G.F. (1970) *J. exp. Med.* **131**, 675.
[53] WEIGLE W.O. (1971) *Clin. exp. Immun.* **9**, 437.
[54] FELDMANN M. & DIENER E. (1971) *Immunology* **21**, 387.
[55] SJÖGREN H.O., HELLSTRÖM I., BANSAL S.E. & HELLSTRÖM K.E. (1971) *Proc. natn. Acad. Sci. U.S.A.* **68**, 1372.
[56] HOWARD J.G., CHRISTIE G.H. & COURTENAY B.M. (1972) *Proc. R. Soc.* (B) **180**, 347.
[57] MCCULLAGH P.J. (1970) *J. exp. Med.* **132**, 916.
[58] BYERS V.S. & SERCARZ E.E. (1970) *J. exp. Med.* **132**, 845.
[59] ANDERSSON J., SJÖBERG O. & MÖLLER G. (1972) Manuscript submitted for publication.
[60] FREI P.C., BENACERRAF B. & THORBECKE G.J. (1965) *Proc. natn. Acad. Sci. U.S.A.* **53**, 20.
[61] BRETSCHER P. & COHN M. (1970) *Science* **169**, 1042.
[62] DRESSER D.W. (1962) *Immunology* **5**, 378.
[63] DIENER E. & ARMSTRONG W.D. (1969) *J. exp. Med.* **129**, 591.
[64] FELDMANN M. (1972) *J. exp. Med.* **135**, 735.
[65] BRITTON S. (1969) *J. exp. Med.* **129**, 591.
[66] HOWARD J.G. (1971) *Ann. N.Y. Acad. Sci.* **181**, 18.
[67] HOWARD J.G., ZOLA H., CHRISTIE G.H. & COURTENAY B.M. (1971) *Immunology* **21**, 535.
[68] DEL GUERICO P. & LEUCHARS E. (1972) *J. Immun.* in press.
[69] MIRANDA J.J. (1972) *Immunology* **23**, 824.
[70] MIRANDA J.J., ZOLA H. & HOWARD J.G. (1972) *Immunology* **23**, 843.
[71] SHELLAM G.R. & NOSSAL G.J.V. (1968) *Immunology* **14**, 273.
[72] LEDERBERG J. (1959) *Science, N.Y.* **129**, 1649.
[73] VON BOEHMER H. & BYRD W.J. (1972) *Nature New Biol.* **235**, 50.
[74] LOUIS J., CHILLER J.M. & WEIGLE W.O. (1972) *Fed. Proc.* **131**, 655.
[75] GERSHON R.K. & KONDO K. (1972) *Immunology* **21**, 903.
[76] NAOR D. & SULITZEANU D. (1967) *Nature, Lond.* **214**, 687.
[77] NAOR D. & SULITZEANU D. (1969) *Int. Archs Allergy* **36**, 112.
[78] ADA G.L. & COOPER M.G. (1971) *Ann. N.Y. Acad. Sci.* **181**, 96.
[79] HUMPHREY J.H. & KELLER H.U. (1970) In *Developmental Aspects of Antibody Formation and Structure*, ed. Sterzl J. & Riha M., p. 485. Academic Press, New York.
[80] RUTISHAUSER U., MILLETTE C.F. & EDELMAN G.M. (1972) *Proc. natn. Acad. Sci. U.S.A.* **69**, 1596.
[81] BRENT L., BROOKS C., LUBLING N. & THOMAS A.V. (1972) *Transplantation* **14**, 382.
[82] BILLINGHAM R.E., BRENT L. & MEDAWAR P.B. (1953) *Nature, Lond.* **172**, 603.

3 · A cellular basis for auto-immunity

J. H. L. PLAYFAIR *Department of Immunology, Middlesex Hospital Medical School, London*

'Is there any other point to which you would wish to draw my attention?'
'To the curious incident of the dog in the night time.'
'The dog did nothing in the night time!'
'That,' remarked Sherlock Holmes, *'was the curious incident.'*

The case of the auto-antibodies is just as curious, the mystery being not why there are so many auto-antibodies but why there aren't *more*. The Great Detective's explanation for the inactivity of the watchdog was that he recognized the intruder as familiar, and the same sort of explanation used to seem vaguely adequate to explain the immunological situation. After all, to a dog all humans must smell fairly similar, and if he can pick out one in a million (incidentally, how does he do it?) it doesn't seem too far-fetched that he can tell my thyroglobulin from his, making antibodies against mine and not his own. But when people *do* start making antibodies against their own antigens, like dogs suddenly biting their master, it poses problems which, with all due respect to numerous theories, I don't think could ever have been completely solved in the state of understanding that prevailed until some six or seven years ago.

Since then, we have had a complete revolution of thinking about antibody production, with the realization that there are two (at least) different sorts of lymphocytes, with many different properties, both involved in practically all antibody responses [1]. The concept of B and T cells is now so entrenched that it is already becoming fashionable to question it. It is of course, only one step in the direction of understanding what immunological cells really do, and there must be many surprises to come, including no doubt a multiplicity of further subdivisions and transitions; however, I cannot see that there is any going back. In this review, I have tried to place auto-immunity in this new context, freely using, mostly without acknowledgement, facts that are reasonably well known and keeping the controversial and unconfirmed ideas for the last section, in which some new hypotheses are put forward that at least have the merit of testability. The problem is definitely not solved; in fact sceptics will probably think it is no nearer solution. All I can say is that it seems a bit clearer to me!

To begin with, and to confine the argument for the moment to auto-antibodies alone—leaving aside the issue of cellular auto-reactivity and indeed the whole question of auto-immunity as *disease*—I ought to briefly describe the multicellular cooperative mechanism of normal antibody formation as it looks at present (at the rate things are going this is probably the part of the review that will be out of date soonest). Antigens bind to preformed antibody receptors on certain lymphocytes (B cells) which then, if antigen and antibody compose the right kind of matrix on their surface proceed to proliferate and secrete antibody of the same type—at least as regards the combining site—as the receptor. These antibodies are coded for by genes many or all of which are inherited. After stimulation, and possibly also before, individual B cells carry receptors of very restricted combining specificity. In the great majority of cases the proper matrix cannot be formed, or proliferation cannot proceed (or both) without the help of other stabilizing structures which may bind other parts of the antigen, most probably at the surface of the macrophage. One important source, but not necessarily the only one, may be the product of other lymphocytes, differentiated in the thymus (T cells). T cells may bind antigen or release antigen-binding factors, or other factors favouring proliferation: the nature of their receptor is not known, but it also has elements of specificity. Though certain large regular antigens can apparently do without T cells, their participation is essential for the formation of the amounts of antibody, particularly IgG, that constitute the normal primary and secondary response. T cells are sensitive to much lower concentrations of antigen than unaided B cells are.

The interaction of at least three different kinds of cell brings a number of new permutations to bear on the auto-antibody problem. For example, B and T cells might both lack receptors for (be 'tolerant' to) all 'self' determinants, either because of absence of the appropriate genes, or by actual elimination of any cell that advertises self-reactivity, or through the presence of factors that block or silence potentially self-reactive cells. Or the tolerance might only affect the T cells, leaving self-reactive B cells willing but powerless for want of a cooperative T cell. Or again, the macrophage might be the decisive cell, by refusing to act as go-between where self-antigens are concerned.

The clues

To help decide among these alternatives, evidence will be called from three experimental situations in which the normal mechanism has been upset namely: (1) **artificial tolerance**, (2) **induced auto-immunity**, and (3) **spontaneous auto-immunity**.

1. ARTIFICIAL TOLERANCE

The classic cases of this were first the accidental induction of unresponsiveness to polysaccharide antigens by high doses, and subsequently the deliberate induction of allogeneic chimeras by neonatal spleen cell injection. Finally large, or ultra-solubilized, doses of proteins joined the list of tolerated antigens. At the risk of over-generalizing one might say that non-thymus-dependent antigens (such as the polysaccharides) tolerize B cells very readily, while proteins, and probably transplantation antigens, tolerize T cells readily and B cells with difficulty. In many cases of 'whole animal' tolerance, only T cells are tolerant.

In the case of the best-known polysaccharide (from type 3 pneumococci) the B-cell tolerance is preceded by some antibody synthesis, and can be rapidly reversed by removing antigen, which squares perfectly with *in vitro*

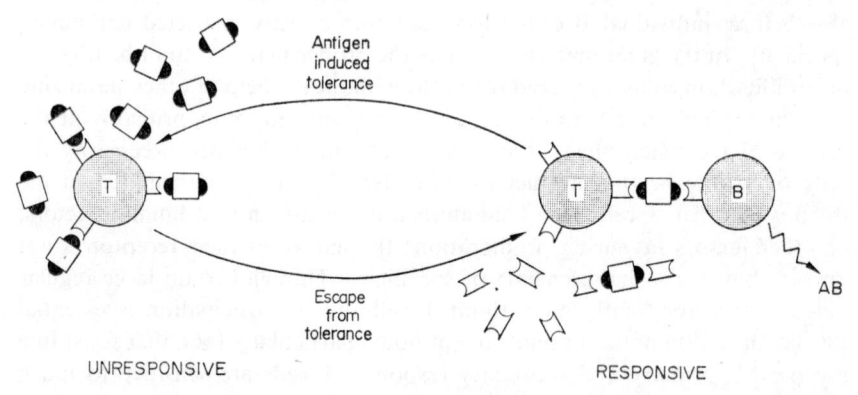

Fig. 3.1. Reversible control by antigen of T-cell reactivity. The white squares with black knobs denote antigen (foreign or self).

evidence for an antigen–antibody matrix of precise proportions as a B-cell 'shut-off' signal. However, another polysaccharide (levan, or polyfructose) is quite different, inducing irreversible tolerance without prior antibody synthesis [2]. Which of these, if either, is the rule and which the exception remains to be seen.

It is likewise in dispute whether T-cell tolerance is due to blocking or elimination. Studies of some apparently 'pure' T-cell reactions, such as stimulation by transplantation antigens (mixed lymphocyte reaction, graft-versus-host disease) suggest that tolerant populations do actually lack cells with the relevant specificity. On the other hand tests involving cytotoxicity *in vitro* have been claimed to reveal auto-reactive cells in transplantation chimeras. One problem is to be certain that these are T cells. Another is that many target cells are known to change their antigenic features rapidly in culture, so that the reaction may be against allo- rather than auto-antigens. The last objection might also apply to experiments in which thymus cells from normal mice have apparently been sensitized to self-antigens *in vitro*. In both cases autologous serum is said to prevent the expression of this latent self-reactivity, and the analogy has been made with the blocking antibodies, which protect tumours from attack by otherwise competent lymphocytes, though it is equally possible that it is soluble antigen in the serum that blocks the T cells (Fig. 3.1). However, this is unlikely to be the case in artificial tolerance, since high doses of antibody to the tolerated antigen will not reverse tolerance [3]. Moreover, a thorough search in transplantation chimeras for factors blocking *in vivo* T-cell responses has so far failed.

In antibody-cooperation experiments, T cells from tolerant animals maintain their unresponsiveness on transfer to antibody-free mice, so here too reversible blocking seems to be ruled out. One aspect that might bear closer study is the difference in the spectrum of reactivity, including anti-self reactivity, between thymus cells and T cells from the spleen, lymph-nodes, etc., since one of the older (and still very reasonable) ideas about T-cell tolerance is that it is induced in the thymus itself, in which case some thymus T cells might be expected to be still at the 'pre-censorship' stage. Of this, more later.

The termination of artificial protein tolerance is of the utmost relevance. The administration of a cross-reacting protein may cause the production of antibodies to the shared (i.e. previously tolerated) antigens, the weaker the cross-reaction (that is, the more the unshared determinants) the better the termination [3]. This irresistibly suggests that the B cells were neither missing nor blocked, but that a deficit somewhere else needed to be by-passed via the new unshared determinants. What has been said about the relative ease of tolerance induction in T cells makes it likely that here it is the T cells which, tolerant to the shared but not the unshared determinants, give the tolerant state its specificity.

2. INDUCED AUTO-IMMUNITY

The many ways of 'terminating natural unresponsiveness' [3] by inducing normal animals to make auto-antibodies, and sometimes destructive lesions, can practically all be interpreted as the administration of exaggerated levels of cross-reacting or 'altered-self' antigens. The damage may be done from within (CCl_4), self antigens may be deliberately modified (aggregated immunoglobulin, virus-coated red cells, substituted thyroglobulin) normal cross-reacting antigens can be used, just as in terminating artfiicial tolerance, or the many-pronged attack of adjuvants may be invoked. Chronic stimulation of the lymphoid system by persistant allogeneic cells probably fits into the same pattern.

By analogy with the termination of artificial tolerance (above), Weigle has argued that the by-passing of a T-cell defect by recruiting other T cells that respond to the unshared determinants on the cross-reacting antigen, is the key to auto-antibody production in these cases. Again, the implication is that B cells capable of making auto-antibodies pre-exist even in normal animals (Fig. 3.2). An interesting prediction of this model, borne out in practice, is that the auto-antibodies will all cross-react with the inducing antigen, but not necessarily with each other.

What is striking about most of these induced auto-antibody responses in normal animals is their transience. A typical 'primary' response consists of IgM only, and several injections, or the aid of adjuvants, are needed to produce high levels of IgG. And even then, the antibody tends to disappear within a few weeks of stopping the injection of antigen. By contrast, the auto-antibodies in chronic spontaneous cases (that is, 'disease') are mainly IgG, and may be present for years. One wonders whether some of the IgM may not turn out to be thymus-independent (Fig. 3.2).

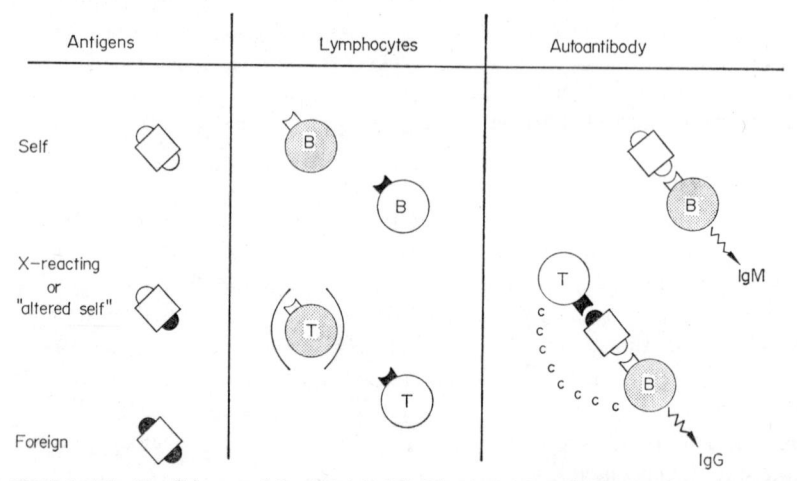

Fig. 3.2. The T-cell bypass (after Weigle [3]). Foreign determinants, and the corresponding receptors, are shown in black, 'self' determinants and receptors in white. Shaded cells are those capable of 'self' recognition. Cells in brackets are postulated to be functionally absent. Cooperation is denoted thus: c c c c c.

The rapidity with which auto-antibodies can appear to at least some intracellular antigens, such as liver mitochondria, makes it virtually certain that, as in artificial tolerance, strict unresponsiveness to these antigens does not exist in the genome, nor in the B cells [4]. Indeed the finding of some IgM auto-antibodies in the absence of any apparent tissue damage has led to the proposal that they have a physiological function in tissue turnover [5].

There are several possible explanations for this difference between the self-limited auto-immune and the ongoing 'disease' auto-antibody response. Persistence of antigen could explain the cases where adjuvants are used, but most theories involve the lymphocytes themselves. Firstly, high affinity memory cells and IgG producing cells might be present but normally be made tolerant, either by excess of antigen (i.e. a lower threshold than the IgM cells) or because some other cell function (T cell or macrophage?)

required for the *avoidance* of tolerance is not forthcoming. Secondly, memory and IgG production may be entirely dependent on T-cell cooperation, which is absent in the case of auto-antigens because of the strictness of T-cell tolerance to self. In this case, auto-antigens would simply resemble any other thymus-independent antigens. Against this idea is the fact that only slightly modified self-antigens do appear in some cases to be rather good carriers for hapten responses. Traditionally this is the role of the T cell, but the development of cooperative mechanisms not dependent on T cells is a possibility (see later).

A third explanation would invoke the 'controlling' T cell. Based on several lines of evidence—the NZB mouse, the thymus-independent antigens, allotype suppression, etc.—the hypothesis has been advanced that some T cells have the function of switching *off* B cells [7]. Though attractive and provocative, this idea raises as many problems as it solves. What recognizes what? One can (just) picture a B cell with a receptor for a *cell-surface* self-antigen stimulating a T cell carrying that antigen and, in so doing, committing suicide, but in the case of B cells with receptors against other self-antigens, it must surely be the T cell that recognizes the B cell. How? The inevitable alteration of a B cell after binding antigen has indeed been put forward as a signal for a T cell, but a signal to *stimulate* antibody production, and it is hard to see exactly the same mechanism, with only a change of antigen, having exactly the opposite effect. There is the possibility, though it smacks rather of the armchair, that the specific T-cell response to a *single* antigenic determinant is in fact always of the 'shut off' type. If so, cooperation with B cells could only result when two determinants are recognized (the 'homospecific exclusion' of Taylor & Iverson [6]), the specific 'stop' signals being overridden by a non-specific 'go' signal (from a T cell reacting against one determinant to a B cell recognizing the other). In the case of auto-antigens, where there is more chance of only a single determinant being recognized, the resulting 'stop' signal might constitute the normal control mechanism. Alternatively, one might simply say that the T cells can recognize and destroy B cells carrying 'forbidden idiotypes', but as demonstrated above, this is certainly not the case with the IgM B cells, which presumably carry the same idiotype that, on an IgG B cell, would be regarded as 'forbidden'. Some possible ways out of this dilemma will be considered in the last section of this essay.

3. SPONTANEOUS AUTO-IMMUNITY

Of the naturally occurring cases of loss of self-tolerance in laboratory animals, two have far outstripped the rest: the NZB mouse and the obese chicken.

NZB mice have been bewildering immunologists for a dozen years with their anti-red cell and anti-nuclear auto-antibodies, and so many other aberrations have since been found that it sometimes looks as though every component of their immune system is totally weird. However, as in some human family studies, there is the catch here that too restricted a 'normal' population is often used for comparison. For example, the tendency of NZB mice to develop myeloma is shared with Balb/c, the production of anti-DNA antibodies is even more marked in some A substrains, spontaneous anti-thymocyte antibodies are found in strain 129, Gross virus lymphoma is far commoner in AKR, low affinity antibody is made by several other strains and so on.

The features of the NZB on which there is a fair consensus are as follows: auto-antibodies are produced against many tissue components, including (inherited) Gross virus, native DNA, red-cell lipoproteins, T cells, cardiolipin. Combined with a tendency to soluble complex formation, the first two or three of these probably account for the glomerulonephritis. Exogenous antigens play little part here. The allo-antibody response has many features of chronic adjuvant treatment, and macrophage function is also increased in a way reminiscent of chronic non-specific stimulation. The cell-mediated immune system declines at an unusually early age in the NZB, but until then is vigorous and relatively resistant to the development of tolerance.

The trouble is that these defects could be arranged in almost any order of cause and effect. Some clues may come from a careful comparison of the age at which various abnormalities are first detectable, and perhaps partly because it is easier to study in very young mice, the cooperative ability of T and B cells in antibody formation has been followed back farthest. In the first week of life only the T cells seem to be abnormal, displaying a resistance to high-dose tolerance that correlates remarkably well with that shown by the animal as a whole. The only other abnormalities reported as early as this also involve the thymus: a histological difference in the epithelial thymic reticulum and the lack of a mysterious factor ('thymosin') in serum, associated with the presence of a normal thymus. Unfortunately, these most provocative findings are also the least confirmed, but they surely focus attention on the thymus as a possible primary source of trouble.

The connection between the thymus and auto-antibodies is not obvious. Neonatal thymectomy sometimes does and sometimes does not precipitate auto-immunity. Perhaps the combination of thymic abnormality (or absence of the thymus) and altered self-antigens (i.e. by virus) is needed. But the lack of T cells does have one striking effect in the NZB—to prolong auto-antibody production by injected spleen cells from old NZB's, themselves already making auto-antibodies. A rather similar result has been derived from experiments with the A/Jax mouse, which spontaneously develops anti-DNA auto-antibodies, apparently inhibitable by the injection of young T cells. These most important findings first introduced the concept of the thymus as a regulator, rather than simply an inducer, of antibody synthesis. One explanation, the controlling T cell, has been referred to; others will be mentioned in the last section of this paper.

The obese chicken, which develops both thyroiditis and thyroid auto-antibodies, bears the same relationship to human organ-specific auto-immunity as the NZB does to the SLE group of diseases. As in the NZB, all the evidence is in favour of a genetic predisposition and against exogenous infection. But there is an important difference at the cellular level. Both the auto-antibodies and the lymphocytic infiltration of the thyroid, which in human disease has often been assumed to belong to the T-cell mediated domain, turn out to be associated with the bursa and not the thymus, The meaning of this discovery has not been fully digested yet, but it does revive interest in the many roles of antibody in tissue destruction. In fact the automatic equation of T cells with cytotoxicity was clearly hasty. Whether the bursa-derived cells themselves become cytotoxic, or merely furnish the anti-target cell antibody for another, non-specific, cell is not yet sorted out. The regulatory role of the thymus in the chicken has not been studied in detail, but thymectomy is said to slightly worsen the thyroiditis and this disease would seem an ideal starting point.

The restriction of a genetically controlled auto-immune disease to a single organ suggests one of two possibilities: an abnormal B cell (mutant antibody) gene or a predisposing weakness in the organ itself. Although a mathematical case has been made out for sequential mutation as a basis for auto-immunity [8], what evidence there is favours the latter idea—including the association in human studies of different organ-specific diseases in the same family, the multigenic segregation of the haemolytic and renal components of the NZB syndrome, and, in the obese chicken itself, a hint that syngeneic thyroid may be more susceptible to damage than allogeneic. Monoclonal auto-antibodies, which the antibody mutation theory would predict, do occur but are by no means the rule.

The general conclusion, then, from these animal models might be that auto-immunity results when several genetic factors come together, some weakening a particular organ and others affecting various parts of the immune system, especially the mechanism by which the thymus enforces tolerance on its progeny.

Summing up

It is now time to briefly appraise the evidence from all three of the experimental situations that have been discussed, and then to suggest a hypothesis that will accommodate them all. Allowing for some simplification and personal bias, it seems to boil down to the following three facts:

B cells able to make antibody against many self-determinants exist in normal animals, and can mount a rapid IgM and a slower IgG response to excess and/or altered self-antigen; T cells reacting with self-determinants do not normally exist, at least outside the thymus. In the absence of T cells, B cells are better able to make ongoing auto-antibody responses, yet in the absence of T cells the normal B cell response to *foreign* antigens is stultified.

Three hypotheses

1   The simplest possible hypothesis would be that auto-immunity is normally held in check by the lack of self-reactive T cells. This should be adequate to

ensure the absence of both IgG auto-antibodies, secondary responses, and T-cell mediated destructive lesions. The system would break down if this T-cell tolerance failed, and, as mentioned earlier, two ways can be envisaged: removal of blocking antigen (Fig. 3.1) or a defect in the postulated thymus censorship mechanism (Fig. 3.3). To take one example, in the NZB a T cell expressing reactivity against the inherited ('self') viral antigens would offer cooperating help to any B cell able to recognize something to which the virus was attached, such as a red cell, or with which it cross-reacted, such as DNA.

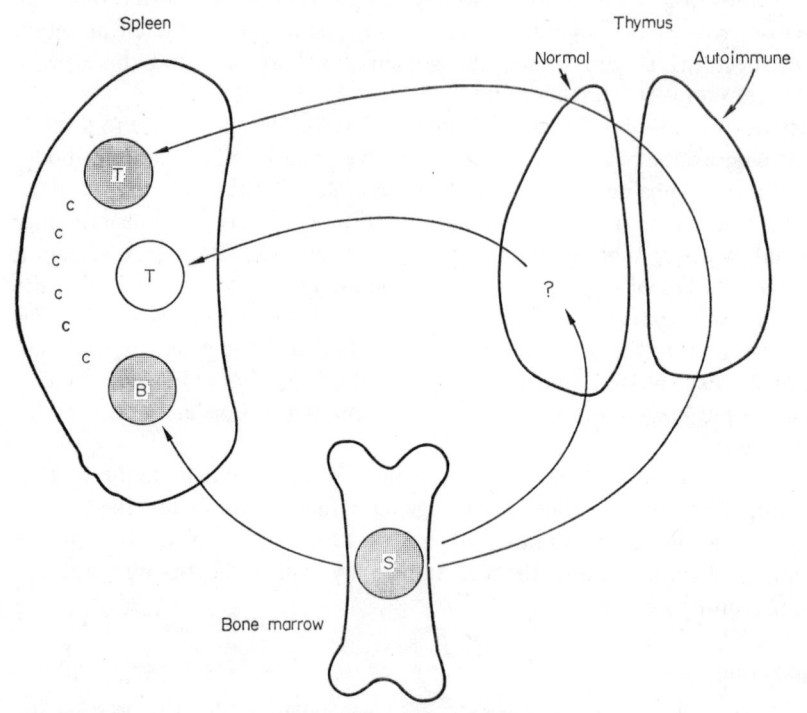

Fig. 3.3. The auto-reactive T cell. S denotes a stem cell: thymus censorship is represented by a question mark. Other symbols as in Fig. 3.2.

This hypothesis, however, is powerless to explain the effect of thymectomy on auto-antibodies. It would predict either no effect (if the peripheral T cells have been normally censored) or a reduction in auto-antibodies (if they haven't). Judging by the NZB, the effect is quite the opposite, and a completely new concept—the controlling T cell—has to be invoked. Also, for what it is worth, NZB mice do not in fact appear to be short of T cells until old age, as judged by the usual T cell markers.

2 One way out of this impasse would be to postulate that the non-T-cell mediated cooperative mechanisms (B cells, carrier antibody, macrophages) might expand in importance, in a compensatory way, when the thymus is absent and, since these are based on antibody—itself not as scrupulously self-tolerant as the T cells—this 'alternative cooperating pathway' would progressively accept self-antigens as carriers, with the inevitable results that self-'haptens' would become progressively more immunogenic (Fig. 3.4). The only evidence that points this way at the moment is the finding that NZB B cells do seem to manage without T cells in the IgM response to foreign red cells better than those of other strains. There is also the interesting discovery that levan (the thymus-independent antigen mentioned earlier) can act as a carrier for DNP, but only in the production of IgM [2].

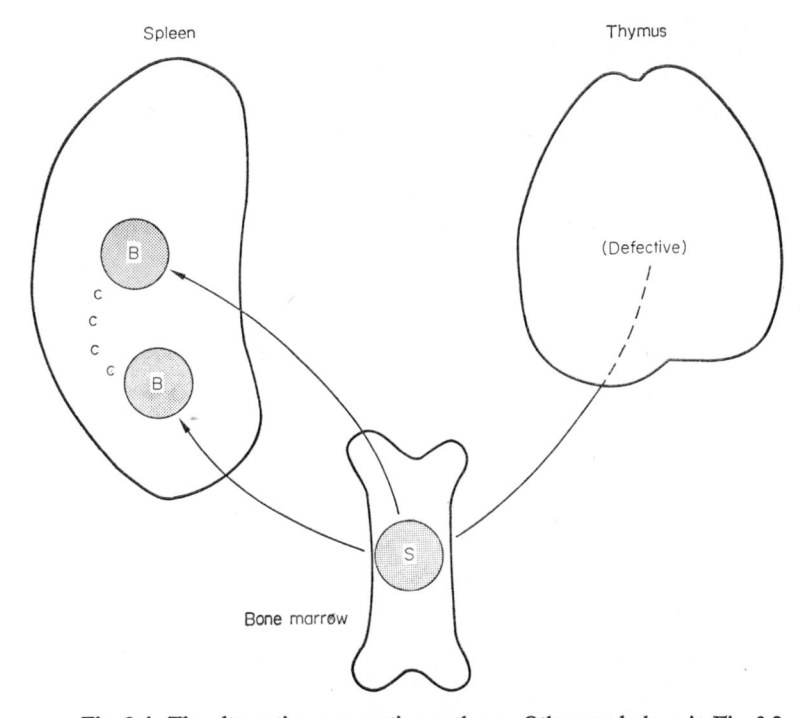

Fig. 3.4. The alternative cooperation pathway. Other symbols as in Fig. 3.2.

3 A completely different solution is to postulate that not only T cell tolerance, but B cell tolerance as well, is maintained by censorship in the thymus, the vital difference being that a T cell, being so to speak *born* in the thymus, is checked for self-reactivity at once, whereas a B cell is only put to the test after antigenic stimulation. In other words, instead of exporting mysterious controlling T cells, the thymus itself does the controlling. (Admittedly, the mechanism of censorship for T cells is also totally mysterious at present, but I feel, like Occam, that one mystery is preferable to two.) Thus the normal population of auto-reactive B cells, produced in the marrow without the benefit of any censorship, can mount a primary response to any antigen their genes permit, foreign or self, but at some stage after this primary response—

either randomly or because of some time-associated surface change—they circulate through the thymus, where the 'forbidden' auto-reactive ones would be eliminated, just as though they were T cells, and the permitted ones allowed out again, perhaps even after a period of expansion. Upon second contact with the self-antigen, new 'pre-censorship' B cells, fresh from the marrow, would merely react again as before, whereas a second contact with the foreign antigen would find an expanded and 'educated' B (as well as T) memory cell population. In the absence of the thymus the elimination of the forbidden B cells would not occur, and a memory population might gradually be built

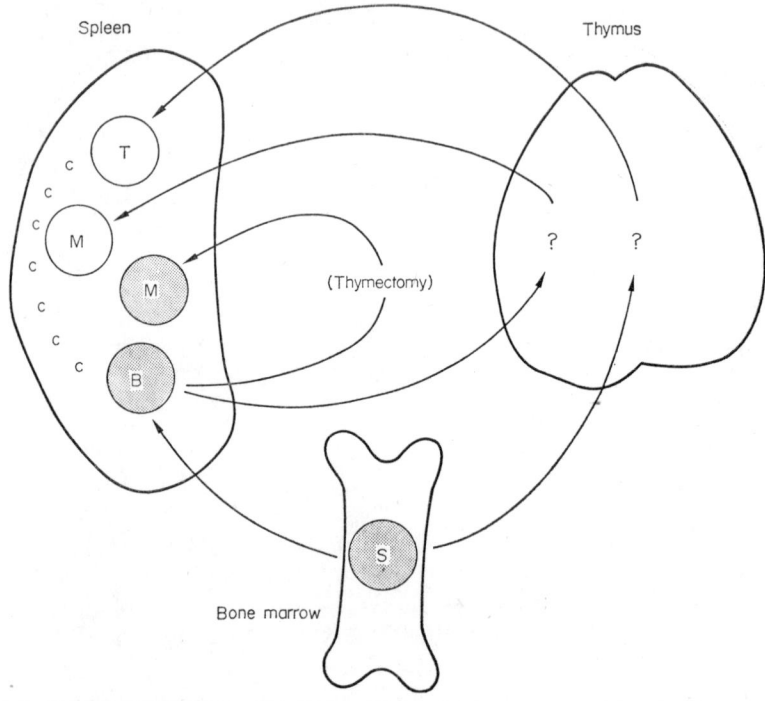

Fig. 3.5. T and B cell censorship by the thymus. M denotes a B memory cell. Other symbols as in Fig. 3.2.

up, especially if there are still some normal T cells present in the periphery, as there will usually be when the thymus has functioned for a time. Also, the permitted B cells might lose their chance of selective expansion in the thymus, and so the tendency will be towards a point where reactivity to self and to non-self will be about equal. Fig. 3.5 illustrates the idea schematically. (It may be added that this hypothesis could meet that of the controlling T cell half-way, by allowing the censorship process to be carried out, albeit less efficiently, outside the thymus—perhaps in the T-cell-dominated areas or 'little thymuses' of the lymph nodes and spleen.)

Several other intriguing predictions follow from this third hypothesis. First, memory resides in B as well as T cells; though once out of favour, this idea is now respectable again, one example being the high affinity antibody that, laboriously selected in the later stages of the primary response, appears promptly in the secondary response. Other examples have come from the study of anti-hapten and anti-sheep cell responses, where B memory cells can be found in the spleen for at least a month. Secondly, B cells should recirculate through the thymus. This is also not as outrageous a notion as it sounds. Careful search of the thymus reveals a few per cent of B cells, and often a lot more in larger, longer-lived animals. And it has recently been claimed that after a primary response to sheep cells, specific B cells can be found in the thymus for a matter of months. The general belief that cells other than marrow do not enter the thymus is based on gross counting of chromosomally labelled cells, where one would probably never detect the small shifts envisaged here. Thirdly, one would predict that thymectomy, even in the adult animal, would impair secondary responses in both B and T populations. Indeed, if the flow of B cells to the thymus could ever be traced to a particular time after the primary response, thymectomy at this time, or even local irradiation, might have the same effect. Luckily these predictions can be tested with great ease.

Either of these three hypotheses would explain the spontaneous animal diseases reasonably well. In the case of the NZB, one would speculate that the primary failure is in the thymus. Hypothesis 1 would require that either the censorship mechanism is the first to fail, or that the NZB T cell develops an undue proneness to reactivity as opposed to tolerance (a shift to the right in Fig. 3.1); in either case the end result is a self-reactive T population. According to hypothesis 2, the 'alternative cooperating pathway' via the B cells themselves takes over, with the results already mentioned. In fact the trouble with this theory is that it might predict a flood of auto-antibodies in *all* thymectomized animals, which is certainly not the general finding.

According to hypothesis 3, B cells will be stimulated by cross-reacting antigens (again, the virus is a possible self-altering agent) by virtue of ordinary T-cell cooperation, forthcoming because of the release of self (virus) reactive T cells before the thymus fails completely. Those B cells responding to the self component (red cells, DNA, etc.) cannot be eliminated by passage through the thymus, and will therefore remain to be stimulated again and again, building up an IgG response and a memory pool. One would like to see a normal thymus graft correcting matters, which has so far not been shown, but it may be that a grafted thymus can never be quite normal. Alternatively, the picture might be further complicated by an element of abnormality in the susceptibility of the B cells to censorship, even by a normal thymus.

In the obese chicken, where destructive lesions and auto-antibody both stem from B cells, the third hypothesis seems to fit best; auto-reactive B cells are not being eliminated, for the same reasons as in the NZB—thymic insufficiency or B-cell-tolerance resistance. Thus a self-reactive population builds up. In this case an abnormality in the thyroid itself may constitute the 'altered-self' stimulus, contrasting with the diffused alteration in the NZB. From the fact that bursectomy prevents both auto-antibody and thyroiditis whilst re-injection of bursa cells restores the latter only, one might hazard the guess that the infiltrating cell is of a type that is less dependent on actual sojourn in the bursa—perhaps a post-bursal cell.

One could go through a long list of human auto-immune syndromes, forcing them to fit one or other of these three hypotheses, but it will be much more convincing to collect further evidence from the animal models. It would be rather typical of science in general if they all turned out to be partly right. Or perhaps none of them will stand up to the test; if so, another theory, even more far-fetched, may have to be considered. To paraphrase the Great Detective again: 'Eliminate all other hypotheses, and the one which remains, however improbable, is the truth.'

References

[1] MITCHISON N.A. (1970) *Transplant. Proc.* **2**, 92.
[2] HOWARD J.G. (1972) *Transplant. Rev.* **8**, 50.
[3] WEIGLE W.O. (1967) *Natural and Acquired Unresponsiveness*. World Publishing Co., Cleveland, Ohio.
[4] WEIR D.M. & ELSON C.J. (1969) *Arthritis Rheum.* **12**, 254.
[5] GRABAR P. (1964) *Molecular and Cellular Basis of Antibody Formation*, p. 621. Czech. Acad. Sci.
[6] TAYLOR R.B. & IVERSON G.M. (1971) *Proc. R. Soc. Lond. B.* **176**, 393.
[7] ALLISON A.C., DENMAN A.M. & BARNES R.D. (1971) *Lancet* ii, 135.
[8] BURNET F.M. (1972) *Auto-immunity and Auto-immune Disease*. Medical and Technical Publishing Co. Ltd., Lancs.

4 · Tumour immunology

N. A. MITCHISON *University College, London*

Tumour immunology is based on the proposition that tumour cells make specific antigens ('TSA', tumour specific antigen), and that these antigens can and should be used for the diagnosis and treatment of cancer. It hopes also to find out whether or not these antigens play a role in the natural history of cancer: for example, it is claimed that people with defects of the lymphoid system run an abnormally high risk of developing cancer, and that these and other kinds of data on cancer epidemiology require an immunological interpretation. Spin-off for other branches of immunology is also expected, in the form of improvement in techniques for assaying cellular immunity and so on. Another sort of spin-off to be hoped for is the provision of markers for cellular differentiation, in the form of differentiation antigens shared in common by normal and tumour cells of the same differentiated type.

These are high aims, and to the intrinsic importance of the subject has been added the attraction of lavish support from the research agencies. Yet one may still inquire why tumour immunology has become the object of such intense interest only recently—after all, in the last few years nothing really revolutionary has come up by way of ideas or technology, and certainly there is little to cite so far by way of clinical success. In the latter respect immunology compares unfavourably with chemotherapy and other less fashionable subjects. I believe that the following circumstances account for the general feeling that immunology is about to fulfil its promise:

(i) The subject has at last outgrown its disreputable history, in the course of which tumour specific antigens got badly confused with transplantation antigens, and outrageous claims were made for serum therapy and diagnosis.

(ii) A decade of rapid progress in cellular immunology must surely lead to applications in clinical medicine, and where if not in cancer?

(iii) For all their successes, neither radiation nor chemotherapy has succeeded in providing a long-term cure for many forms of cancer, whereas immunity, being more natural, promises to do so.

(iv) Thanks to the Hellströms we have seen in rapid succession first the

demonstration of lymphocytes cytotoxic to tumour cells present in individuals bearing a tumour, then specific serum factors which block the activity of these lymphocytes, and finally procedures which counteract the blocking factors.
(v) Thanks largely to Matthé, the first glimmers of success in the immunotherapy of cancer in man have been seen.

I propose now to discuss, in succession, the problems of cancer prevention, detection, and cure. Let us begin with the matter of prevention: what hope is there of reducing the incidence of cancer by large-scale immunization of normal people? However far-fetched this question may seem, it serves at least to raise the interesting problem of the distinction between unique and common tumour-specific antigens. For obviously, since one cannot predict what kind of tumour an individual may develop, the success of prior immunization must depend on the vaccine and the prospective tumour sharing antigens in common. The first tumour-specific antigens that were discovered in the carcinogen-induced tumours of mice turned out to be highly specific for individual tumours; indeed so unsuccessful has been the search for cross-reactions among these tumours that their antigens can provisionally be regarded as unique. On theoretical grounds this conclusion seems unacceptable, and a certain amount of rather unfruitful debate has gone on over the question whether these 'unique' antigens result from mutations in structural genes or from stable re-arrangements of elements already coded for in the normal cell. At any rate, it looked to start with as though the uniqueness of the tumour-specific antigens would impede immunization and diagnosis. This fear, it now turns out, may not be justified, for at least two kinds of common antigen—common to a range of tumours—have since been discovered: the virus-induced and oncofoetal antigens.

Of these, the virus-induced are the better understood. The oncogenic viruses divide into two quite distinct groups, DNA viruses and RNA viruses, each with a characteristic set of antigens. Tumours induced by DNA viruses have a cell surface antigen which is quite distinct from those of the virus, but which nevertheless can be assumed to be coded for by the virus rather than the cell, for the same antigen is found on the cells of tumours induced by a given virus irrespective of the host species. Tumours induced by RNA virus also have a common surface antigen, but in this case the antigen seems to be identical with that found on the viral envelope. The tumour cell sheds RNA virus and in the early stages of budding the viral envelope can be clearly seen in the electron microscope to run continuously into the cell membrane. Virus envelope antigen can be detected also in other areas of the membrane, where budding does not occur, so that one gains the impression that the elements of the envelope are inserted irregularly into the cell surface and then gathered together over the virus core. The consequence of this is that antibody to the virus can easily lyse the cell, and that a response to the virus is mainly responsible for protective immunity to the tumour. This proposition requires some qualification however; it is supported by studies on the specificity of humoral antibody, and by comparisons made between virus-shedding and non-shedding lines of tumour cells, but it is not entirely in accord with the most recent data (including my own) on the specificity of cell-mediated immunity.

Until recently the RNA viruses were stronger candidates than DNA viruses for the role of causative agent in human cancer, and as such have attracted a great deal of attention. This is partly for negative reasons: no DNA virus is definitely known to induce tumours in its native host among mammals. In a positive way, RNA viruses have been identified as causing leukaemias and mammary carcinoma in mice. Particles resembling the mouse mammary carcinoma virus have been found in human milk, and circumstantial evidence links their occurrence there with cancer of the breast. Epidemiological data are also compatible with a viral origin for childhood leukaemia. It is natural therefore to prepare a programme, as has been done by Huebner and his colleagues at the National Cancer Institute in Washington, which runs roughly as follows. First of all, the techniques for identifying and handling the RNA virus would be worked out in the convenient mouse systems. Next, a search would be carried out for human oncogenic RNA viruses. In this search immunology would have a part to play: in order to carry conviction as a human oncogenic agent, any virus should contain the intergroup-specific antigen of the known mammalian RNA-oncogenic viruses (shared in common by the cat, hamster and mouse leukaemia viruses), but should lack the group-specific antigens of the known laboratory viruses (otherwise contamination would be suspected). Other criteria would presumably operate as well: to judge from the mouse model, one could expect a true human oncogenic virus to induce tumours in other primates, although inoculation into immuno-suppressed animals or into foetuses might be necessary. Once such virus had been isolated, the next stage in the programme could commence. Large amounts of virus will be grown up *in vitro* in order to produce a vaccine made up of attenuated or inactivated virus. Finally, the vaccine would be tested, first in primates and then in man.

So clear is this programme and so determined is the group in Washington that there is little point in arguing—one can only wish them luck. Indeed the programme is already under way, and at least one virus has been identified which satisfies the immunological criteria just mentioned. It is no criticism of the programme to point out that RNA viruses only *cause* cancer in a very restricted sense; the cells of mice vertically infected with leukaemia virus are bathed in virus particles, yet less than one cell in a million becomes malignant, under circumstances which are not, but ought to be understood. The point is that if we are able to eliminate the virus before the malignant transformation has occurred, we may be able to prevent the transformation without under-standing much about its nature. It is more pertinent to emphasize that the DNA viruses, and experience which is being gained with their immuno-logical control in animals, ought not to be neglected. For example, Marek's disease of poultry, which is caused by a DNA virus, and in which something like lymphosarcoma develops, is at present the object of a very large-scale vaccination trial.

Before leaving the question of vaccination we might return again to the other type of antigen common to a range of tumours, the oncofoetal antigens. Can we imagine them being used for vaccination? At first sight the suggestion seems absurd, for these antigens although wide-spread are generally extremely weak, and have almost completely failed to confer protective immunity against transplanted tumours in some quite stringent tests. Nevertheless, I do not think the suggestion is entirely hopeless, if one is willing to accept TL (the thymus leukaemia antigen of mice) as a general case. In normal non-tumour tissue this antigen has a restricted distribution, being present only on thymus lymphocytes. It is present neither on stem cells of the lymphoid line prior to their entry into the thymus, nor on mature T cells which have passed out into the peripheral lymphoid tissue; indeed it appears to be lost during the process of maturation within the thymus, shortly before the lymphocytes emerge. Thus it puts in an appearance only during a limited and well-defined stage of differentiation of a restricted group of cells. Fortunately, strains of mice exist which lack TL—TL-negative strains—so that the antigen is not only a differentiation antigen, but also a differentiation allo-antigen. This permits allo-antisera to be raised which in turn enable the distribution and location of the antigen to be defined with precision. With the aid of these allo-antisera the antigen has been identified not only within the thymus but also on many leukaemic cells. If one is willing to accept an antigen which is present during a limited stage of development as a sort of foetal antigen, TL provides an instance of an oncofoetal antigen which is present only in a restricted group of normal cells. Other oncofoetal antigens can then also be expected to show a limited distribution in normal tissue; one can hope that stronger immunity can be raised to such antigens by using the appropriate foetal tissue, than if unselected foetal tissue is used in bulk. The study of oncofoetal antigens is still at an early stage, and the hunt for restricted antigens of the postulated type has not yet begun.

One has to admit certain qualifications to the argument. The TL system shows certain features which one can hardly expect to prove typical of oncofoetal antigens. For example, it appears on leukaemic cells of TL-negative as well as TL-positive strains. Normally this is taken to mean that the negative strains have a normal structural gene plus a defective control gene, which is by-passed in leukaemic cells. An alternative possibility is that TL is virus-coded, and that the segregation of TL is due to the segregation of an IR gene (immune response gene) or other sort of gene which determines susceptibility to virus infection. This interpretation may seem far-fetched, but it is precisely what has been proposed for the G_{IX} antigen (an antigen related to Gross virus infection, which is controlled by a locus on chromosome IX of the mouse), and TL and G_{IX} have embarrassing similarities.

I shall turn now to my second topic, cancer detection by immunological methods. Here the greatest success has been achieved with those tumours which release a product which can be identified in the blood. The prime examples here are tumours of the colon, which secrete a carcino-embryonic antigen (referred to as CEA), and hepatomas, which secrete alpha-foetal-protein. CEA, which is a glycoprotein, and alpha-foetal-protein, can both be identified by heterologous antisera in radio-immunoassays. Work with CEA has proceeded to the point where mass screening of the normal human population can at least be imagined, although at present the consensus of opinion holds that this would not be justified mainly because of the high incidence of false positives. In the meanwhile the test has useful clinical applications, for example in the identification or metastases after surgery. From a general standpoint, the merits and drawbacks of these kinds of tests are becoming clear. Their chief merit is that a well-defined product is present in solution in plasma, and this enables classical immunochemical methods to be applied. One major drawback is that they seem unlikely to provide a general solution to the problem of cancer detection: we have little reason to hope that other tumours will release equally characteristic products. Another is that the products seem to be characteristic not of tumour cells as such, but of a particular kind of cell in a proliferative or inflammatory phase. For this reason it looks as though false positives are going to be not just an incidental nuisance, but a basic feature of this kind of test. At the same time one has to admit that it is only because work on CEA has gone ahead so well that we are able to recognize these limitations: no doubt other approaches will be subject to similar qualifications when they have reached the same stage.

The approach to detection which I think looks most promising at present is the use of long-term tumour cell lines. The general plan is to use these cell lines to monitor for heightened reactivity in lymphocytes taken from apparently normal people. Obviously there are all sorts of problems, of which the most prominent is the extent to which different tumours of the same type can be expected to cross-react with a single cell line. Animal experiments with carcinogen-induced tumours are not encouraging in this respect. Cytotoxic lymphocytes taken from human cancer patients seem to cross-react to a much greater extent: perhaps the best example is a long-term line of bladder carcinoma cells, which has for nearly a hundred *in vitro* passages retained susceptibility to lysis by lymphocytes from a large panel of patients with this particular form of tumour, but not other lymphocytes. Comparable examples could be cited from melanoma, and from certain sarcomas. The reason for this discrepancy between animals and man has not been identified. One possibility is that the human cross-reactions reflect common viral antigens, but this seems less and less likely as the number of groups of cross-reactive tumours increases. One wonders whether the tempo of tumour development may be relevant: the animal studies have been made with relatively rapidly developing tumours.

The attractive thing about research on long-term cell lines, and immunological reactivity towards them, is that what needs doing is clear and feasible. We need to know more about the cell biology of growth from the initial explant: how much selection occurs, what decides whether fibroblasts will overgrow, how can we influence these processes, when should the cells be cloned? We need to know how to cope with heavily infected tumour tissue: does transplantation into the B-mouse* provide a useful intermediate stage?

* A mouse effectively deprived of thymus dependent (T) lymphocytes.

We need to know more about infection of lines with C-particle viruses: should routine radio-immunoassay for the group-specific (GS) antigen be performed at intervals, can one select with anti-type-specific sera, do the infections originate in the laboratory, do they matter from an immunological standpoint? We need to know for how long lines can be passaged without losing the relevant antigens, and more about the technology and practical operation of frozen cell banks. Above all we need to know how best to assay the reactivity of the lymphocytes: can they be stored successfully prior to test, should they be fractionated, does it pay to add auxiliary tests, will the isotope assays which are coming into vogue replace the older visual methods?

Having stated a point of view, let me give briefly my opinion about the cytopherometer test for cancer, however distasteful it may seem to deal in generalities with something so controversial and potentially so important. The test is based on the discovery that antigen triggers lymphocytes to release one or more factors which then interact non-specifically with macrophages. The classical method of demonstrating this interaction is to show that the macrophages become less able to migrate—hence the term migration inhibition factor (MIF). It has been found that macrophages exposed to these factor(s) also migrate more slowly in an electric field. Caspary & Field have used this slowing, which can be measured in a cytopherometer, to demonstrate lymphocyte reactivity of many cancer patients towards a common cancer antigen (a basic protein thought to be present in the cell membrane). Although the importance of this claim can be recognized immediately, the test has not come into wide use. Perhaps there has not been enough time yet, but one is put off by the difficulty which has been encountered in repeating an apparently simple test, and the lack of understanding of the underlying mechanisms. However the test *has* been repeated successfully by at least one other group.

My opinion is that we need to know more about how this test works before trying to decide whether or not it is more sensitive than other ones. We assume that cytotoxicity and colony-inhibition tests, skin tests of delayed hypersensitivity, migration inhibition tests, and the cytopherometer test are all aimed at the same thing: detecting T cells which have been triggered by tumour-specific antigens. In order to make a rational choice among competing tests, we surely need to know whether the same subpopulation of lymphocytes is active in all tests, whether a cell which secretes factors necessarily becomes cytotoxic, whether there is a succession of activities, and so on. These are difficult matters to investigate, because the factors secreted by T cells are so obscure. Indeed, if anything, confusion is growing, not only because early optimism about the chemistry of MIF has given way to the appalling notion that activated T cells liberate at least a dozen different proteins (based on biosynthetic labelling), but also because T cells now seem to secrete a specific factor as well! How eagerly one hopes for a satisfactory method of enumerating individual T cells activated by tumour-specific antigens.

Let us turn to our third and last topic, the immunotherapy of cancer.

Immunotherapy so far has much less to offer than immunodiagnosis in terms of practical achievements, so we can do little more than guess at how developments will proceed. The general idea is clear enough: the responses to tumour-specific antigens which are at present too weak to eliminate the tumour will somehow be amplified up to the level at which elimination is obtained. Two sorts of strategy aiming at this goal seem at present to be worth exploring, those which seek simply to increase the response, and those which seek rather to depress factors which block the natural response. For the time being neither strategy is likely to be implemented except as a more or less minor adjunct to surgery, chemotherapy, or radiation. What we are likely to see is more of the kind of trial which has been introduced by Matthé, in which leukaemia patients are brought into remission by chemotherapy, and then treated by immunotherapy in the hope of delaying relapse. To treat initially by immunological procedures would be morally unacceptable at the present time, and would in any case be unlikely to work; for experimental studies on animals have shown that immunological mechanisms which can cope with small tumour masses can easily be swamped by larger ones.

Immunotherapy has been thoroughly studied in experimental tumour systems, particularly with the transplantable tumours of mice and guinea-pigs. In most but not all cases it has proved possible to immunize against the tumour, provided that immunization commences either before transplantation or at least before the tumour has attained much size; in a few cases, particularly in the guinea-pig, immunization is even possible at later stages. In the course of these studies it has become clear that immunization can be achieved most easily (a) by using inactivated or attenuated tumour cells, and (b) by combining specific immunization of this kind with non-specific stimulation of the immune response (i.e. by using adjuvants). One can therefore see a broad avenue of approach to immunotherapy in man involving a combination of specific and non-specific stimulation of the immune response by established methods. This is not of course to under-rate the contribution which fundamental immunology has still to make in this area: we are still distressingly ignorant, for example, of the mode of action of even the oldest established adjuvants—although one might reasonably argue that at this stage empirical screening of adjuvants in human trials has more to offer than analysis in animal models.

Has fundamental immunology something more to contribute? Can one hope to exploit recent progress in order to improve cancer immunotherapy? There are two recent discoveries which look to me particularly promising. One of these is the help which one lymphocyte can give another in making an immune response. (This matter is also discussed elsewhere in the present volume by Nossall and Playfair.) To summarize the present state of knowledge, there appear to be two mechanisms by which T lymphocytes help the response of B lymphocytes. One is by presentation: receptors on the surface of the T lymphocytes pick up a multideterminant antigen by one determinant (the helper determinant), and present it in the form of a matrix which facilitates its binding, via other determinants (the inducing determinant) to surface receptors on B lymphocytes. The matrix is probably constructed not on the T lymphocyte itself but on the surface of a macrophage which adsorbs the shed T lymphocyte receptor in complex with antigen. The other is by means of non-specific factors secreted by stimulated T lymphocytes: these agent(s), none of which has yet been isolated, are thought to stimulate the proliferation and differentiation to mature immunological activity of other lymphocytes.

Thus far the most refined analysis of these two mechanisms has been performed *in vitro*, and we are less clear about their importance, and relative roles *in vivo*. My impression is that presentation is probably more important in most *in vivo* responses, although factors can help under certain circumstances, particularly of vigorous immunological stimulation (e.g. the allogeneic effect). It is likely that determinants on particular types of carrier may need one form of help rather than the other. Perhaps the greatest area of uncertainty lies in the application of these mechanisms to helping the response of T lymphocytes. Thus far the analysis has been worked out almost entirely with B lymphocytes as the recipients of help, and attempts to demonstrate help for T lymphocytes have yielded equivocal results. Since T-lymphocyte-mediated cytotoxicity (in the traditional terminology, cell-mediated immunity) appears to be crucial for destroying tumour cells, this is a question of great importance. My guess, based (a) on the flimsy evidence available at present, and (b) on the latest version of the presentation hypothesis involving a matrix on the macrophage surface, is that help of the same sort can be used by T lymphocytes. What is clear is that the new knowledge of help from T to B lymphocytes gives moral encouragement to investigating other forms of response amplification.

Have we any direct evidence that help from T lymphocytes can be exploited for cancer immunotherapy? Lindenmann & Klein found that Ehrlich tumour TSA incorporated into the influenza virus envelope (or at least associated with that envelope) evokes a particularly powerful immune response. Their findings have been confirmed and extended by studies on the immunogenicity of TSA from SV-40 transformed cells associated with influenza virus. Both these studies involved cell membrane preparations, rather than intact tumour cells. In an extensive study of TSA associated with Newcastle Disease Virus (NDV), my colleague Dr P.C.L.Beverley, in collaboration with Dr D.Tyrell and Dr R.Levinthal, finds that virus infected tumour cells are not more immunogenic than irradiated cells. If, however, cell membranes rather than intact cells are employed, the expected increase in immunogenicity is obtained. In these experiments the favourable effect obtained on the survival of subsequent tumour transplants is small in comparison with the effect obtained on the humoral response to TSA; this, it might be argued, augurs ill for help for T-cell-mediated responses. Nevertheless it is encouraging that both recent studies could demonstrate appreciable increases in the effectiveness of immunotherapy, attributable to cooperation between lymphocytes.

New light on the nature of helper determinants on the cell surface has been cast by the recent work of Iverson & Lindenmann on the response of mice to the liver auto-antigen F. The humoral response to this antigen is cooperative, in the sense that it appears to require help from T lymphocytes reacting to a cell surface allo-antigen. The helper allo-antigen turns out not to be H-2. Thus the strongest surface antigens are not necessarily the best helpers. Why this should be the case is not clear: possibly the dense distribution of H-2 over the cell results in steric hindrance. Evidently we still have much to learn about what makes a good helper determinant.

The second discovery which I believe may contribute to cancer immunotherapy is that T and B lymphocytes have different requirements for triggering. The ability to activate differentially the two arms of the immune response gives us the power to control immunization with much greater precision than ever before, although the implications of this new capability for cancer immunotherapy are not clear in detail. If anything, matters are at present more obscure than a few years ago, when the Hellströms had taught us to write the simple equation cellular immunity = good, humoral antibody = bad. The evidence now suggests that in at least some instances, notably melanoma, blocking factors are antigens, rather than antibody. Indeed, humoral antibody may play a beneficial role by inactivity tumour-specific antigen which has been liberated into the plasma, although it may also prevent small antigenic fragments from being rapidly cleared out of the body; the matter simply is not clear. But whatever the final relevance of humoral immunity in immunity to tumours, there can be little doubt that we shall need to be able to modulate the response during immunotherapy.

When one actually comes to write down the rules for differential T/B triggering, matters are again not as clear as one would wish, or as one had hoped a year or two ago that they would be. One can put it, a trifle paradoxically, as follows. For the soluble antigens and mitogens the rules are fairly consistent. High concentrations of antigen favour triggering B lymphocytes, not only for immunity but also for tolerance; highly aggregated antigens and mitogens also favour B lymphocytes, presumably because their repeating determinants make up a favourable matrix; reduction in the affinity of individual determinants favour T lymphocyte triggering—witness the consequence of aceto-acetylating flagellin. But now what happens when we try to apply these rules to cell surface antigens? Perhaps the clearest comparison is between H-2 determinants, as presented to the immune system in their natural matrix on the surface of allogeneic cells, or as a papain-solubilized low molecular weight extract. Here the aggregated antigen induces a response in both types of lymphocyte, while the low molecular weight material triggers differentially B cells (as shown perhaps most clearly in the induction of tolerance). This is exactly the opposite of what one could expect from the work with soluble antigens.

Let me not conclude on a note of pessimism. What matters is that these problems have been identified: much better to have a clear-cut difference, and the tools available for further work, than vague uncertainty. Surely a productive period lies ahead in which the rules of basic cellular immunology will be applied to the response to tumours.

Further reading

[1] BURNET F.M., PREHN R.T., LAPPÉ M.A., MCKHANN C.F., JAGARLAMOODY S.M., WALFORD R.L., SMITH G.S., WATERS H., STARZL T.E., PENN I., PUTNAM G.W., GROTH C.C., HALGRIMSON C.G. & BRITTON S. (1972) Immunological surveillance against neoplasia. *Transplant. Rev.* 7.
[2] HELLSTRÖM K.E., SJÖGREN H., MATHÉ G. & SMITH R. (1971) In *Progress in Immunology*, ed. Amos B. Academic Press, N.Y.
[3] OLD L.J., BOYSE E.A., GEERING G. & OETTGEN H.F. (1968) Serological approaches to the study of cancer in animals and man. *Cancer Res.* **28**, 1288.
[4] MITCHISON N.A. (1973) Immunology of cancer in animals. In *Clinical Aspects of Immunology*, eds. Gell P.G.H. & Coombs R.R.A. 3rd edition. Blackwell, Oxford.